Path to Freedom

100 Transformative Worksheets for Substance
Abuse Recovery

Micah Helene Olson

ISBN- 978-1-923238-56-5

Jstone Publishing

Disclaimer

The names and scenarios depicted in this book are purely for illustrative purposes only. Any resemblance to actual persons, living or dead, or actual events is purely coincidental. The scenarios are designed to demonstrate the application of the book's principles in various life situations and should not be interpreted as specific advice for personal issues. Readers are encouraged to consult with a qualified healthcare provider for personalized advice and treatment options.

Preface

Welcome to " Path to Freedom: 100 Transformative Worksheets for Substance Abuse Recovery." This book is a comprehensive resource designed to support individuals on their journey to overcoming substance abuse and reclaiming their lives. Substance abuse is a complex and challenging issue that affects millions of people worldwide, impacting not only the individual but also their families, communities, and society as a whole. Recognizing the need for accessible and effective tools to aid in the recovery process, we have compiled a collection of worksheets that draw from evidence-based practices and therapeutic techniques.

Each section of this book is carefully crafted to address key aspects of the recovery journey, offering guidance, reflection, and practical exercises to empower individuals to take control of their lives and make positive changes. From self-reflection and goal setting to coping strategies and relapse prevention, these worksheets are designed to be used in conjunction with professional treatment and support services.

As you embark on your journey to recovery, it is important to remember that change is possible, and you are not alone. Recovery is a process that requires dedication, perseverance, and support. This book is intended to serve as a companion on your path to wellness, providing you with the tools and resources you need to navigate the challenges of substance abuse recovery.

We would like to express our gratitude to the therapists, counselors, and individuals with lived experience who contributed to the development of this book. Their expertise and insights have been invaluable in creating a resource that is both practical and empowering.

Whether you are just beginning your recovery journey or are further along in the process, we hope that "" Path to Freedom: Transformative Worksheets for Substance Abuse Recovery " will serve as a valuable resource and guide on your path to healing and transformation.

With warm regards,

Micah Helene Olson

Table of Contents

Introduction

Brief overview of substance abuse and its impact

Substance abuse refers to the harmful or hazardous use of psychoactive substances, including alcohol and illicit drugs, which can lead to dependence, addiction, and a range of physical, psychological, and social consequences. Substance abuse often involves the repeated use of substances despite negative consequences, such as health problems, impaired functioning, strained relationships, legal issues, and financial difficulties.

The impact of substance abuse can be profound and far-reaching, affecting individuals, families, communities, and society. Some of the key impacts of substance abuse include:

1. **Physical Health Effects:** Substance abuse can lead to a variety of physical health problems, including liver disease, cardiovascular issues, respiratory problems, neurological damage, infectious diseases (such as HIV/AIDS and hepatitis), and overdose-related injuries or fatalities.
2. **Mental Health Effects:** Substance abuse is often associated with mental health disorders, such as depression, anxiety, psychosis, and mood disorders. Substance use can exacerbate existing mental health conditions and increase the risk of developing new ones.

3. **Social and Interpersonal Consequences:** Substance abuse can strain relationships with family members, friends, and coworkers, leading to conflicts, breakdowns in communication, and social isolation. It can also impair social functioning, making it difficult to maintain employment, fulfill social roles, and engage in productive activities.

4. **Legal and Criminal Justice Issues:** Substance abuse can result in legal problems, including arrests, fines, probation, and incarceration, particularly if individuals engage in illegal activities to support their substance use or if their substance use leads to impaired driving or other criminal behaviors.

5. **Financial Burden:** Substance abuse can impose a significant financial burden on individuals and society, including costs related to purchasing substances, healthcare expenses for treatment and rehabilitation, legal fees, lost productivity, and damage to property or public infrastructure.

6. **Risk of Addiction and Dependence:** Continued substance abuse can lead to addiction, a chronic, relapsing disorder characterized by compulsive drug-seeking and use despite negative consequences. Addiction can profoundly impact brain function, behavior, and decision-making, making it challenging to stop using substances without professional help.

Overall, substance abuse is a complex and multifaceted issue that requires comprehensive prevention, intervention, and treatment strategies to address effectively. By addressing the underlying factors contributing to substance abuse, providing access to evidence-based treatment and support services, and promoting healthy behaviors and coping mechanisms, it is possible to mitigate the impact of substance abuse and improve outcomes for individuals and communities affected by this issue.

Importance of recovery worksheets in the rehabilitation process

Recovery worksheets play a crucial role in the rehabilitation process for individuals recovering from substance abuse and addiction. Here's why they are important:

1. **Self-Reflection and Insight:** Recovery worksheets encourage individuals to reflect on their thoughts, emotions, behaviors, and experiences related to substance abuse. By engaging in self-reflection exercises, individuals gain insight into the underlying factors contributing to their addiction, identify triggers and patterns of behavior, and explore their motivations for change.

2. **Goal Setting and Planning:** Worksheets provide a structured framework for setting and planning goals related to recovery. By helping individuals clarify their values, aspirations, and priorities, recovery worksheets enable them to set realistic and achievable goals for sobriety, personal growth,

and overall well-being. This process empowers individuals to take ownership of their recovery journey and develop concrete action plans for achieving their goals.

3. **Skill Building and Coping Strategies:** Worksheets introduce individuals to a variety of coping skills, strategies, and techniques for managing cravings, coping with stress, and navigating challenges in recovery. By practicing these skills through guided exercises, individuals build resilience, develop healthy coping mechanisms, and strengthen their ability to effectively manage triggers and temptations without resorting to substance use.

4. **Increased Self-Awareness and Accountability:** Engaging in recovery worksheets promotes self-awareness, accountability, and responsibility for one's actions and choices. By documenting their progress, setbacks, and reflections, individuals gain a deeper understanding of themselves, their behaviors, and the impact of substance abuse on their lives. This awareness fosters a sense of accountability for making positive changes and staying committed to the recovery process.

5. **Enhanced Communication and Expression:** Worksheets provide a structured platform for individuals to communicate their thoughts, feelings, and experiences in a safe and supportive environment. By expressing themselves through written exercises, individuals can articulate their concerns, fears, and aspirations, facilitating honest

and open communication with therapists, peers, and support networks.

6. **Promotion of Positive Change and Growth:** Recovery worksheets support individuals in making positive changes and fostering personal growth throughout the recovery journey. By engaging in meaningful self-reflection, goal setting, and skill building activities, individuals cultivate a sense of empowerment, resilience, and hope for the future. This process of positive change contributes to long-term sobriety, improved well-being, and a fulfilling life in recovery.

Overall, recovery worksheets serve as valuable tools for promoting self-discovery, goal achievement, skill development, and personal transformation in the rehabilitation process. By incorporating these worksheets into treatment programs and therapy sessions, individuals can gain valuable insights, develop essential coping skills, and take proactive steps toward lasting recovery from substance abuse and addiction.

Section 1: Self-Reflection Worksheets

These self-reflection worksheets are designed to encourage introspection, insight, and personal growth as individuals navigate the journey of substance abuse recovery. Encourage users to engage with the worksheets thoughtfully and regularly, seeking support from therapists, support groups, or trusted loved ones as needed.

Identifying Triggers Worksheet

Description: This worksheet is designed to help you recognize the specific situations, emotions, people, or places that trigger the urge to use substances. By identifying your triggers, you can develop strategies to avoid or cope with them effectively.

Time: Allocate 15-20 minutes for this activity.

Activities:

1. **Reflect on Past Instances:** Take a few moments to reflect on past instances of substance use. Recall situations where you experienced a strong urge to use substances.
2. **Identify Triggers:** Write down the specific triggers associated with each instance. These may include social gatherings, stressful situations, certain emotions (such as loneliness or anxiety), specific people, or places.
3. **Rate the Intensity:** Rate the intensity of each trigger on a scale from 1 to 10, with 1 being least intense and 10 being most intense.
4. **Reflect on Significance:** Consider the significance of each trigger. Even seemingly insignificant triggers should be noted, as they may contribute to your overall pattern of substance use.

5. **Be Honest:** Be honest with yourself as you complete the worksheet. Don't dismiss any triggers, no matter how small they may seem.

Guidance: Take your time to recall each trigger vividly. Be honest with yourself and write down any triggers that come to mind, even if they seem insignificant. Remember that identifying triggers is the first step towards effectively managing them and preventing relapse. Use this worksheet as an opportunity for self-discovery and insight into your patterns of substance use.

Understanding Cravings Worksheet

Description: This worksheet aims to help you understand the sensations and thoughts you experience when craving substances. By describing these feelings in detail, you can develop awareness and coping strategies to manage cravings effectively.

Time: Set aside 15-20 minutes for this activity.

Activities:

1. **Reflect on Cravings:** Take a moment to reflect on past experiences of craving substances. Recall the physical sensations and mental patterns associated with these cravings.
2. **Describe Sensations:** Write down the physical sensations you typically experience when craving substances. These may include a racing heart, sweaty palms, or tension in specific muscle groups.

3. **Explore Mental Patterns:** Describe the thoughts and emotions that accompany cravings. Notice any obsessive thoughts about using substances or feelings of desperation or anxiety.
4. **Rate Intensity:** Rate the intensity of your cravings on a scale from 1 to 10, with 1 being mild and 10 being overwhelming.
5. **Reflect on Triggers:** Consider the triggers that commonly precede cravings, such as stress, boredom, or exposure to certain cues.

Guidance: Pay attention to both physical sensations and mental patterns when reflecting on cravings. This awareness can help you develop effective coping strategies to manage cravings when they arise. Remember that cravings are a natural part of the recovery process, and by understanding them, you can empower yourself to resist the urge to use substances.

Exploring Motivation Worksheet

Description: This worksheet encourages you to consider the reasons why you want to overcome substance abuse. By identifying both short-term and long-term motivations for recovery, you can stay focused and committed to your goals.

Time: Allocate 15-20 minutes for this activity.

Activities:

1. **Reflect on Goals:** Think about your goals for recovery, both short-term and long-term. Consider what you hope to achieve by overcoming substance abuse.
2. **Identify Motivations:** Write down the reasons why you want to stop using substances. These may include improving your health, repairing relationships, pursuing career or educational goals, or reclaiming control of your life.
3. **Consider Values:** Reflect on how achieving sobriety aligns with your core values and beliefs. Consider how substance abuse may conflict with these values.
4. **Visualize Success:** Take a moment to visualize what your life will look like when you have successfully overcome substance abuse. Imagine yourself living a fulfilling and meaningful life free from the grip of addiction.

Guidance: Reflect on how achieving sobriety aligns with your values and aspirations. Keep this list handy as a source of inspiration during challenging moments. Remember that your motivations for recovery may evolve over time, so revisit this worksheet regularly to stay connected to your goals.

Assessing Risky Situations Worksheet

Description: This worksheet prompts you to identify situations or environments where you're more likely to be tempted to use substances. By recognizing high-risk situations, you can plan ahead and implement strategies to avoid relapse.

Time: Set aside 15-20 minutes for this activity.

Activities:

1. **List High-Risk Situations:** Write down situations, environments, or triggers that increase your risk of using substances. These may include social gatherings where alcohol is present, stressful situations, encountering old drinking or using buddies, or feeling lonely or bored.
2. **Rate Risk Level:** Rate the level of risk associated with each situation on a scale from 1 to 10, with 1 being low risk and 10 being high risk.
3. **Identify Warning Signs:** Consider the warning signs that indicate you may be at risk of relapse in each situation. These may include physical cravings, heightened stress levels, or changes in mood or behavior.
4. **Develop Strategies:** Brainstorm strategies for avoiding or coping with high-risk situations. These may include avoiding triggers when possible, practicing stress-reduction techniques, or reaching

out to a supportive friend or family member for help.

Guidance: Be honest about potential triggers, even if they involve activities or places you enjoy. Recognizing high-risk situations empowers you to plan ahead and avoid relapse. Use this worksheet to develop a proactive relapse prevention plan tailored to your unique triggers and vulnerabilities.

Recognizing Patterns Worksheet

Description: This worksheet encourages you to review your past substance use history and identify any recurring patterns or cycles. By recognizing these patterns, you can anticipate challenges and develop proactive coping strategies.

Time: Allocate 15-20 minutes for this activity.

Activities:

1. **Review Past Substance Use:** Reflect on your past experiences of substance use. Consider when, where, and why you typically used substances.
2. **Identify Patterns:** Look for common themes or triggers that precede substance use. These may include specific times of day, social situations, emotional states, or thoughts and beliefs.
3. **Consider Consequences:** Reflect on the consequences of these patterns, both positive and negative. Consider how these patterns may have

impacted your relationships, health, finances, and overall well-being.

4. **Develop Coping Strategies:** Brainstorm coping strategies for managing these patterns effectively. Consider how you can disrupt the cycle of behavior and replace substance use with healthier alternatives.

Guidance: Look for common themes or triggers that precede substance use. Understanding these patterns can help you anticipate challenges and develop proactive coping strategies. Use this worksheet as a tool for self-discovery and insight into your patterns of behavior.

Exploring Consequences Worksheet

Description: This worksheet prompts you to reflect on the negative consequences of substance abuse in various areas of your life. By acknowledging the full impact of substance use, you can strengthen your commitment to change.

Time: Set aside 15-20 minutes for this activity.

Activities:

1. **Reflect on Consequences:** Consider the short-term and long-term consequences of substance abuse in various areas of your life, including relationships, health, finances, and work or school.

2. **List Consequences:** Write down specific examples of negative consequences you have experienced as a result of substance use. These may include

strained relationships, health problems, legal issues, financial difficulties, or academic or occupational setbacks.

3. **Consider Emotional Impact:** Reflect on the emotional toll of these consequences. Consider how substance abuse may have contributed to feelings of guilt, shame, or regret.

4. **Visualize Change:** Take a moment to visualize what your life will look like when you have successfully overcome substance abuse. Imagine yourself free from the burden of addiction, enjoying healthier relationships, improved health, financial stability, and a sense of fulfillment and purpose.

Guidance: Consider both the short-term and long-term effects of substance use. Acknowledging the full impact can strengthen your commitment to change. Use this worksheet as a tool for motivation and reinforcement of your decision to pursue sobriety.

Identifying Support Systems Worksheet

Description: This worksheet prompts you to list individuals or resources in your life that offer support and encouragement for your recovery journey. By cultivating a strong support network, you can enhance your chances of sustained recovery.

Time: Allocate 15-20 minutes for this activity.

Activities:

1. **Reflect on Support:** Think about the people or resources in your life that have offered support and encouragement for your recovery journey.
2. **List Support Systems:** Write down the names of individuals who have been supportive of your efforts to overcome substance abuse. This may include family members, friends, mentors, therapists, support group members, or community organizations.
3. **Consider Types of Support:** Reflect on the types of support each individual or resource provides. This may include emotional support, practical assistance, accountability, guidance, or a listening ear.
4. **Express Gratitude:** Take a moment to express gratitude for the support you have received. Consider reaching out to these individuals to thank them for their role in your recovery journey.

Guidance: Think beyond immediate family and friends to include support groups, therapists, or community organizations. Cultivating a strong support network is essential for sustained recovery. Use this worksheet to recognize and appreciate the people and resources that contribute to your journey toward sobriety.

Exploring Values Worksheet

Description: This worksheet encourages you to reflect on your core values and beliefs and consider how substance use aligns or conflicts with these values. By clarifying your values, you can find purpose and direction in your recovery journey.

Time: Set aside 15-20 minutes for this activity.

Activities:

1. **Reflect on Values:** Consider the core values and beliefs that are important to you. These may include honesty, integrity, health, family, relationships, personal growth, spirituality, or contributing to society.
2. **Consider Alignment:** Reflect on how substance use aligns or conflicts with your values. Consider whether substance use supports or undermines your ability to live in accordance with your values.
3. **Clarify Priorities:** Identify which values are most important to you and how you can prioritize them in your life. Consider how sobriety can help you live in alignment with your values and pursue what matters most to you.
4. **Set Goals:** Use your values as a guide for setting goals and making decisions in your recovery journey. Consider how your values can inform your actions and choices moving forward.

Guidance: Clarifying your values can provide a sense of purpose and direction in your recovery journey. Use this worksheet to reconnect with what truly matters to you and align your actions with your values.

Identifying Coping Strategies Worksheet

Description: This worksheet prompts you to brainstorm healthy coping strategies that you can use to manage stress, cravings, and challenging emotions. By exploring a range of coping techniques, you can find what works best for you.

Time: Allocate 15-20 minutes for this activity.

Activities:

1. **Brainstorm Coping Strategies:** Take a few moments to brainstorm a list of healthy coping strategies that you can use to manage stress, cravings, and challenging emotions. Consider a wide range of options, including physical activities, relaxation techniques, creative outlets, social support, and self-care practices.
2. **Explore Options:** Reflect on the coping strategies you have used in the past and how effective they were. Consider which strategies you found most helpful and which ones you would like to explore further.
3. **Experiment:** Experiment with different coping techniques to see what works best for you. Try out different strategies in various situations and take

note of which ones help you feel better and more resilient.

4. **Develop a Toolkit:** Compile a list of your preferred coping strategies to create a personalized toolkit for managing stress and cravings. Keep this list handy so you can easily access it when you need support.

Guidance: Explore a range of coping techniques, such as exercise, mindfulness, creative activities, or reaching out to supportive individuals. Experiment with different strategies to find what works best for you. Remember that building a diverse repertoire of coping skills can strengthen your resilience and enhance your ability to navigate challenges in recovery.

Setting Boundaries Worksheet

Description: This worksheet encourages you to reflect on boundaries that you need to set in order to protect your sobriety. By establishing clear boundaries, you can maintain a healthy lifestyle and prioritize your well-being.

Time: Set aside 15-20 minutes for this activity.

Activities:

1. **Reflect on Boundaries:** Take a few moments to reflect on the boundaries that you need to set in order to protect your sobriety. Consider situations, relationships, or behaviors that may pose a risk to your recovery.

2. **Identify Triggers:** Identify potential triggers or situations that you need to limit or avoid in order to maintain your sobriety. These may include social gatherings where substances are present, relationships with individuals who enable or encourage substance use, or environments where you feel tempted to use substances.

3. **Establish Boundaries:** Establish clear boundaries for yourself in these areas. Be assertive in communicating your boundaries to others and stick to them consistently.

4. **Plan Ahead:** Consider how you will enforce your boundaries and handle situations where they may be challenged. Develop strategies for maintaining your boundaries in difficult or tempting situations.

Guidance: Establishing clear boundaries is crucial for maintaining a healthy lifestyle. Be assertive in communicating your boundaries to others and prioritize your well-being. Use this worksheet to identify potential triggers and establish proactive strategies for protecting your sobriety.

Exploring Triggers Worksheet

Description: This worksheet encourages reflection on the underlying emotions and thoughts associated with identified triggers for substance use. By understanding the root causes of triggers, individuals can develop more effective coping strategies to manage them.

Time: Allocate 15-20 minutes for this activity.

Activities:

1. **Reflect on Triggers:** Review the triggers you identified in the previous worksheet. Take a moment to think about why these situations or stimuli provoke the urge to use substances.
2. **Explore Emotions and Thoughts:** Dive deeper into the emotional and psychological aspects of each trigger. Consider the feelings, thoughts, memories, or associations that arise in these situations.
3. **Write Down Insights:** Write down your reflections on each trigger, including any insights or revelations about why they have such a powerful effect on you.
4. **Consider Root Causes:** Reflect on any underlying issues or past experiences that may contribute to your reactions to these triggers. Consider how these triggers may be linked to unmet emotional needs, trauma, or coping mechanisms.

Guidance: Take your time to explore the emotional and psychological aspects of your triggers. Understanding the root causes can empower you to develop more effective coping strategies. Use this worksheet as an opportunity for self-discovery and insight into your patterns of substance use.

Self-Assessment of Substance Use Patterns Worksheet

Description: This worksheet prompts individuals to evaluate their patterns of substance use, including frequency, quantity, and situations in which they are most likely to use. By conducting a thorough self-assessment, individuals can make informed decisions about their recovery journey.

Time: Set aside 15-20 minutes for this activity.

Activities:

1. **Reflect on Substance Use Patterns:** Take a moment to reflect on your history of substance use. Consider how often you use substances, the quantity consumed, and the contexts in which you typically use.
2. **Assess Frequency:** Evaluate the frequency of your substance use over time. Consider whether your use has increased, decreased, or remained consistent.
3. **Assess Quantity:** Reflect on the amount of substances you typically consume during a session. Consider whether you have experienced tolerance or escalation in your usage.
4. **Identify Situations:** Identify the situations or environments in which you are most likely to use substances. These may include social gatherings, specific times of day, or emotional states.

5. **Consider Consequences:** Reflect on the consequences of your substance use, both positive and negative. Consider how your use has affected your health, relationships, work or school performance, and overall well-being.

Guidance: Be honest and thorough in your assessment of your substance use patterns. Recognizing the extent of your use can help you make informed decisions about your recovery journey. Use this worksheet as a tool for self-reflection and gaining clarity on your relationship with substances.

Exploring Coping Mechanisms Worksheet

Description: This worksheet encourages individuals to identify past and current coping mechanisms used to deal with stress, pain, or difficult emotions. By assessing the effectiveness and consequences of these coping strategies, individuals can explore healthier alternatives.

Time: Allocate 15-20 minutes for this activity.

Activities:

1. **Reflect on Coping Mechanisms:** Think about the strategies you have used in the past to cope with stress, pain, or difficult emotions. Consider both healthy and unhealthy coping mechanisms.
2. **Identify Strategies:** Write down the coping mechanisms you have relied on, including behaviors, thoughts, or actions. Consider how

31

these strategies have helped you cope in the short term.

3. **Assess Effectiveness:** Evaluate the effectiveness of each coping mechanism in addressing your needs and managing distress. Consider whether these strategies have had any negative consequences in the long term.

4. **Explore Alternatives:** Brainstorm healthier alternatives to replace maladaptive coping mechanisms. Consider strategies that promote long-term well-being and support your recovery goals.

5. **Create a Plan:** Develop a plan for implementing these new coping strategies in your daily life. Consider how you can integrate them into your routine and use them proactively to manage stress and difficult emotions.

Guidance: Assess the effectiveness and long-term consequences of each coping strategy. Explore healthier alternatives to replace maladaptive coping mechanisms. Use this worksheet as a tool for building a repertoire of healthy coping skills that support your recovery journey.

Exploring Family Dynamics Worksheet

Description: This worksheet encourages reflection on the role of family dynamics in an individual's substance use history. By considering family patterns, communication styles, and relationships, individuals can gain insight into how family dynamics may have influenced their behavior and attitudes toward substance use.

Time: Set aside 15-20 minutes for this activity.

Activities:

1. **Reflect on Family History:** Take a moment to reflect on your family history, including patterns of substance use, communication styles, and relationship dynamics.
2. **Identify Influences:** Consider how family dynamics may have influenced your behavior and attitudes toward substance use. Reflect on whether there were any family members who used substances or enabled substance use.
3. **Explore Communication Styles:** Reflect on the communication styles within your family. Consider whether open communication and emotional expression were encouraged or discouraged.
4. **Consider Roles:** Reflect on the roles you and other family members played within the family system. Consider whether these roles contributed to patterns of substance use or influenced your perceptions of yourself and others.
5. **Evaluate Impact:** Consider how family dynamics may have impacted your behavior, attitudes, and coping mechanisms. Reflect on any positive or negative influences your family had on your substance use history.

Guidance: Recognize how family dynamics may have influenced your behavior and attitudes toward substance use. This awareness can inform your recovery process and interactions with family members. Use this worksheet as an opportunity for self-reflection and understanding the role of family in your recovery journey.

Exploring Peer Influence Worksheet

Description: This worksheet encourages reflection on the influence of peers or social circles on an individual's substance use. By identifying individuals who may have encouraged or enabled substance use, individuals can evaluate the impact of peer pressure and consider strategies for setting boundaries.

Time: Allocate 15-20 minutes for this activity.

Activities:

1. **Reflect on Peer Influence:** Think about the people you spend time with and how they may influence your behavior, particularly regarding substance use. Consider whether certain friends or social circles have encouraged or enabled substance use.

2. **Identify Influential Individuals:** Write down the names of individuals who have influenced your substance use behavior. Consider whether these individuals have been supportive of your recovery efforts or whether they have contributed to challenges or setbacks.

3. **Evaluate Impact:** Reflect on the impact of peer pressure on your decisions related to substance use. Consider whether you have felt pressured to use substances in certain social situations or whether peer influence has affected your ability to maintain sobriety.
4. **Set Boundaries:** Consider strategies for setting boundaries with peers who may encourage or enable substance use. Reflect on how you can assertively communicate your boundaries and prioritize your recovery goals.
5. **Seek Supportive Relationships:** Identify individuals or social circles that are supportive of your recovery journey. Consider spending more time with individuals who encourage healthy behaviors and provide positive reinforcement.

Guidance: Evaluate the impact of peer pressure on your decisions related to substance use. Consider strategies for setting boundaries and surrounding yourself with supportive peers. Use this worksheet as an opportunity to reflect on the influence of peers on your recovery journey and identify ways to cultivate a supportive social network.

Exploring Identity and Self-Image Worksheet

Description: This worksheet prompts individuals to reflect on how substance use has affected their sense of identity and self-image. By exploring the impact of substance abuse on self-esteem and self-concept, individuals can cultivate self-compassion and acceptance as they work toward a healthier self-image.

Time: Set aside 15-20 minutes for this activity.

Activities:

1. **Reflect on Self-Image:** Take a moment to reflect on how substance use has influenced your self-image and sense of identity. Consider whether substance abuse has affected your self-esteem, self-confidence, or perception of yourself.
2. **Explore Discrepancies:** Reflect on any discrepancies between your true self and the self-image shaped by substance use. Consider whether substance abuse has led you to act in ways that are inconsistent with your values or aspirations.
3. **Practice Self-Compassion:** Cultivate self-compassion and acceptance as you explore the impact of substance abuse on your self-image. Recognize that substance abuse does not define your worth as a person and that recovery is a journey of growth and self-discovery.
4. **Set Positive Affirmations:** Write down positive affirmations or statements that affirm your worth and potential outside of substance use. Use these affirmations to counteract negative self-talk and reinforce a healthier self-image.
5. **Celebrate Progress:** Celebrate your progress in recovery and acknowledge the steps you are taking toward a healthier, more authentic self-image.

Recognize that change is possible and that you have the power to shape your identity on your own terms.

Guidance: Explore the impact of substance use on your sense of identity and self-image. Cultivate self-compassion and acceptance as you work toward a healthier self-concept. Use this worksheet as a tool for self-reflection and empowerment in your recovery journey.0

Exploring Coping Strategies for Urges Worksheet

Description: This worksheet focuses on brainstorming coping strategies specifically tailored to manage urges and cravings for substances. By identifying effective techniques, individuals can develop a personalized toolkit for managing urges effectively.

Time: Allocate 15-20 minutes for this activity.

Activities:

1. **Identify Urges:** Reflect on the urges and cravings you experience for substances. Consider when these urges typically arise and the intensity of each urge.
2. **Brainstorm Coping Strategies:** Brainstorm a list of coping strategies that you can use to manage urges and cravings. Consider a variety of techniques, such as distraction, relaxation exercises, or engaging in enjoyable activities.

3. **Experiment with Techniques:** Experiment with different coping techniques to see what works best for you. Try out each strategy in different situations and take note of its effectiveness in reducing cravings.
4. **Develop a Toolkit:** Compile a list of your preferred coping strategies to create a personalized toolkit for managing urges. Keep this list handy so you can easily access it when cravings arise.
5. **Practice Coping Skills:** Practice using your coping skills regularly, even when you're not experiencing cravings. Building familiarity with these techniques can make them more effective when you need them most.

Guidance: Experiment with a variety of coping techniques, such as distraction, relaxation exercises, or engaging in enjoyable activities. Develop a personalized toolkit for managing urges effectively. Use this worksheet as a guide for building resilience and strengthening your ability to resist cravings in recovery.

Exploring Values and Goals Alignment Worksheet

Description: This worksheet prompts individuals to reflect on whether their current behaviors and goals align with their core values and aspirations. By realigning actions with values, individuals can pursue fulfilling objectives in recovery.

Time: Set aside 15-20 minutes for this activity.

Activities:

1. **Reflect on Values:** Consider your core values, beliefs, and aspirations. Reflect on what matters most to you in life and the principles that guide your decisions and actions.
2. **Assess Alignment:** Reflect on whether your current behaviors and goals align with your core values. Consider whether your actions are consistent with the person you aspire to be.
3. **Identify Misalignment:** Identify any areas where there is a discrepancy between your values and your actions. Reflect on behaviors or goals that may conflict with your values or detract from your sense of purpose.
4. **Set Intentions:** Set intentions for aligning your behaviors and goals with your core values. Identify specific actions you can take to live in accordance with your values and pursue meaningful objectives in recovery.
5. **Track Progress:** Keep track of your progress in realigning your actions with your values. Celebrate successes and adjust your approach as needed to stay true to your values in recovery.

Guidance: Reflect on how substance use may have hindered your progress toward meaningful goals. Use this worksheet to realign your actions with your values and pursue fulfilling objectives in recovery. Use this worksheet as a tool for self-reflection and setting intentions for living a values-based life in recovery.

Exploring Trauma and Emotional Pain Worksheet

Description: This worksheet prompts individuals to reflect on past traumas or emotional pain that may have contributed to their substance use. By acknowledging the impact of unresolved trauma, individuals can seek support to address underlying emotional wounds.

Time: Allocate 15-20 minutes for this activity.

Activities:

1. **Reflect on Trauma:** Reflect on any past traumas or emotional pain that you have experienced. Consider how these experiences have affected your emotional well-being and coping mechanisms.
2. **Acknowledge Impact:** Acknowledge the impact of unresolved trauma on your mental health and substance use. Consider whether trauma may have contributed to the development of addictive behaviors or coping strategies.
3. **Seek Support:** Consider seeking support from therapy or counseling to address underlying emotional wounds. Reflect on the benefits of processing trauma in a safe and supportive environment.
4. **Practice Self-Compassion:** Practice self-compassion as you explore the impact of trauma on your life.

Recognize that healing from trauma takes time and effort, and that it's okay to seek help when needed.

5. **Explore Healing Techniques:** Explore healing techniques such as mindfulness, self-soothing activities, or expressive arts therapy. Experiment with different approaches to find what works best for you in addressing trauma and emotional pain.

Guidance: Acknowledge the impact of unresolved trauma on your mental health and coping mechanisms. Seek support from therapy or counseling to address underlying emotional wounds. Use this worksheet as a tool for self-reflection and exploring avenues for healing in recovery.

Exploring Healthy Coping Strategies Worksheet

Description: This worksheet prompts individuals to identify and explore healthy coping strategies that provide comfort and support without resorting to substance use. By focusing on building a diverse repertoire of coping skills, individuals can strengthen their resilience in recovery.

Time: Set aside 15-20 minutes for this activity.

Activities:

1. **Brainstorm Coping Strategies:** Brainstorm a list of healthy coping strategies that you can use to manage stress, emotions, and cravings. Consider a variety of techniques, such as physical activities, creative outlets, and social support networks.

2. **Identify Personal Preferences:** Consider which coping strategies resonate most with you. Reflect on activities or techniques that you enjoy and find effective in managing stress and emotions.
3. **Experiment with Techniques:** Experiment with different coping strategies to see what works best for you. Try out each technique in different situations and take note of its effectiveness in reducing stress and enhancing well-being.
4. **Develop a Coping Toolkit:** Compile a list of your preferred coping strategies to create a personalized toolkit for managing stress and cravings. Keep this list handy so you can easily access it when needed.
5. **Practice Self-Care:** Prioritize self-care practices as an essential component of your recovery journey. Incorporate activities that nurture your physical, emotional, and spiritual health into your daily routine.

Guidance: Focus on building a diverse repertoire of coping skills, including physical activities, creative outlets, and social support networks. Practice these strategies regularly to strengthen your resilience and enhance your ability to navigate challenges in recovery. Use this worksheet as a guide for exploring and implementing healthy coping strategies in your life.

Exploring Patterns of Rationalization Worksheet

Description: This worksheet encourages individuals to reflect on the ways in which they justify or rationalize substance use to themselves and others. By increasing awareness of thought patterns that perpetuate addictive behaviors, individuals can challenge irrational beliefs and excuses.

Time: Allocate 15-20 minutes for this activity.

Activities:

1. **Reflect on Rationalizations:** Reflect on the ways in which you justify or rationalize substance use to yourself and others. Consider common excuses or justifications that you have used to justify your behavior.
2. **Identify Thought Patterns:** Identify thought patterns that perpetuate addictive behaviors. Reflect on any irrational beliefs or cognitive distortions that influence your attitudes toward substance use.
3. **Challenge Rationalizations:** Challenge irrational beliefs and excuses that enable continued substance abuse. Consider the evidence against these rationalizations and the consequences of believing them.
4. **Develop Alternative Perspectives:** Develop alternative perspectives that support your recovery goals. Consider more rational and empowering

ways of thinking about substance use and its impact on your life.

5. **Practice Self-Reflection:** Practice self-reflection regularly to increase awareness of your thought patterns and rationalizations. Use journaling or mindfulness techniques to observe your thoughts without judgment.

Guidance: Increase awareness of thought patterns that perpetuate addictive behaviors. Challenge irrational beliefs and excuses that enable continued substance abuse. Use this worksheet as a tool for self-reflection and developing more rational perspectives on substance use in recovery.

Exploring Personal Strengths Worksheet

Description: This worksheet prompts individuals to identify their personal strengths, talents, and qualities that can support their recovery journey. By acknowledging their strengths, individuals can leverage them as resources for overcoming challenges in recovery.

Time: Set aside 15-20 minutes for this activity.

Activities:

1. **Identify Strengths:** Reflect on your personal strengths, talents, and qualities. Consider the characteristics that have helped you overcome challenges in the past and navigate difficult situations.

2. **Celebrate Achievements:** Celebrate your achievements and successes in recovery. Reflect on the progress you have made and the obstacles you have overcome along the way.
3. **Acknowledge Resilience:** Acknowledge the resilience and determination that you possess. Recognize that recovery is a journey of growth and self-discovery, and that you have the strength to overcome challenges.
4. **Leverage Strengths:** Consider how you can leverage your strengths to support your recovery journey. Identify ways in which you can apply your strengths to overcome challenges and achieve your goals.
5. **Set Positive Intentions:** Set positive intentions for using your strengths to overcome obstacles in recovery. Commit to harnessing your inner resources and staying resilient in the face of adversity.

Guidance: Celebrate your strengths and acknowledge the resilience and determination that you possess. Leverage these strengths as resources for overcoming challenges in recovery. Use this worksheet as a tool for self-reflection and empowerment in your recovery journey.

Exploring Personal Triggers Worksheet

Description: This worksheet prompts individuals to identify internal triggers, such as emotions, thoughts, or physiological sensations, that contribute to cravings or relapse. By developing strategies for managing internal triggers, individuals can strengthen their ability to maintain sobriety.

Time: Allocate 15-20 minutes for this activity.

Activities:

1. **Identify Internal Triggers:** Reflect on the internal triggers that contribute to cravings or relapse. Consider the emotions, thoughts, memories, or physical sensations that often precede substance use.
2. **Explore Triggers:** Dive deeper into the specific triggers you have identified. Consider the circumstances or contexts in which these internal triggers tend to arise.
3. **Reflect on Associations:** Reflect on any associations or patterns you notice between internal triggers and substance use. Consider whether certain emotions or thoughts consistently precede cravings.
4. **Develop Coping Strategies:** Develop strategies for managing internal triggers when they arise. Consider mindfulness practices, emotional regulation techniques, or self-soothing activities as potential coping mechanisms.
5. **Practice Awareness:** Practice awareness of your internal triggers on a regular basis. Use journaling or mindfulness techniques to observe your thoughts and emotions without judgment.

Guidance: Develop strategies for managing internal triggers, such as mindfulness practices, emotional regulation techniques, or self-soothing activities. Use this worksheet as a tool for increasing awareness of internal triggers and developing effective coping strategies in recovery.

Exploring Relationships with Substances Worksheet

Description: This worksheet prompts individuals to reflect on their relationship with substances, including how it has evolved over time and its impact on various areas of their lives. By exploring healthier alternatives for meeting needs traditionally fulfilled by substances, individuals can cultivate a more balanced and fulfilling lifestyle.

Time: Set aside 15-20 minutes for this activity.

Activities:

1. **Reflect on Relationship:** Reflect on your relationship with substances, including how it has evolved over time. Consider how your attitudes, behaviors, and perceptions of substances have changed.
2. **Explore Impact:** Reflect on the impact of substance use on various areas of your life, such as relationships, work or school, physical health, and emotional well-being. Consider both positive and negative aspects of your relationship with substances.

3. **Identify Needs:** Reflect on the needs that substances have traditionally fulfilled for you, such as coping with stress, managing emotions, or seeking pleasure. Consider healthier alternatives for meeting these needs.
4. **Consider Consequences:** Reflect on the consequences of continued substance use on your life. Consider the physical, emotional, social, and legal repercussions of substance abuse.
5. **Explore Alternatives:** Explore healthier alternatives for meeting the needs traditionally fulfilled by substances. Consider activities, hobbies, relationships, and coping strategies that promote well-being and fulfillment without relying on substances.

Guidance: Consider the role that substances have played in coping with stress, managing emotions, and seeking pleasure. Explore healthier alternatives for meeting these needs. Use this worksheet as a tool for reflecting on your relationship with substances and identifying ways to cultivate a healthier lifestyle in recovery.

Exploring Boundaries with Others Worksheet

Description: This worksheet prompts individuals to evaluate their boundaries in relationships and interactions with others, particularly concerning substance use. By establishing clear boundaries to protect their sobriety and well-being, individuals can cultivate healthier relationships and environments in recovery.

Time: Allocate 15-20 minutes for this activity.

Activities:

1. **Reflect on Boundaries:** Reflect on the boundaries you need to set in relationships and interactions with others, particularly concerning substance use. Consider situations, behaviors, or environments that may threaten your sobriety or well-being.
2. **Identify Boundaries:** Identify specific boundaries that you need to establish to protect your recovery journey. Consider boundaries related to substance use, communication, time management, and personal space.
3. **Communicate Boundaries:** Develop strategies for communicating your boundaries assertively and effectively. Consider how you can express your needs and expectations clearly and respectfully in relationships.
4. **Enforce Boundaries:** Reflect on ways to enforce your boundaries consistently and assertively. Consider strategies for maintaining boundaries in different situations and addressing boundary violations when they occur.
5. **Seek Support:** Seek support from supportive individuals, such as friends, family members, or therapists, in establishing and maintaining boundaries. Consider joining support groups or seeking professional guidance if you need additional assistance.

Guidance: Establish clear boundaries to protect your sobriety and well-being in relationships and interactions with others. Communicate your boundaries assertively and enforce them consistently. Use this worksheet as a tool for reflecting on your boundaries and cultivating healthier relationships and environments in recovery.

Exploring Emotions Worksheet

Description: This worksheet prompts individuals to reflect on the range of emotions they experience and how they relate to substance use. By practicing identifying and regulating emotions without relying on substances, individuals can develop healthier coping strategies and emotional resilience in recovery.

Time: Set aside 15-20 minutes for this activity.

Activities:

1. **Reflect on Emotions:** Reflect on the range of emotions you experience on a regular basis. Consider both positive and negative emotions, as well as the intensity and duration of each emotion.
2. **Identify Emotions:** Practice identifying and labeling emotions accurately. Use a feelings chart or list of emotions to help you articulate and name your emotional experiences.
3. **Explore Triggers:** Reflect on the situations, thoughts, or events that trigger different emotions for you. Consider how these triggers influence your emotional responses and coping strategies.

4. **Practice Regulation:** Explore healthy ways to express and regulate emotions without turning to substances. Consider relaxation techniques, mindfulness practices, physical activity, or creative outlets as ways to cope with difficult emotions.
5. **Develop Coping Strategies:** Develop a personalized toolkit of coping strategies for managing emotions in recovery. Experiment with different techniques and strategies to find what works best for you in different situations.

Guidance: Practice identifying and regulating emotions without relying on substances. Develop a personalized toolkit of coping strategies for managing emotions in recovery. Use this worksheet as a tool for increasing awareness of your emotions and developing healthier coping strategies in recovery.

Exploring Coping Strategies for Stress Worksheet

Description: This worksheet prompts individuals to identify stressors in their lives and brainstorm healthy coping strategies to manage stress effectively. By experimenting with stress-reduction techniques such as exercise, relaxation exercises, or engaging in hobbies, individuals can develop a personalized stress management plan to support their sobriety.

Time: Allocate 15-20 minutes for this activity.

Activities:

1. **Identify Stressors:** Reflect on the stressors in your life that may contribute to feelings of tension or overwhelm. Consider both external stressors, such as work or relationship challenges, and internal stressors, such as negative thought patterns or self-imposed pressure.

2. **Brainstorm Coping Strategies:** Brainstorm a list of healthy coping strategies that can help you manage stress effectively. Consider techniques such as physical exercise, deep breathing exercises, meditation, journaling, or spending time in nature.

3. **Experiment with Techniques:** Experiment with different stress-reduction techniques to determine which ones work best for you. Try out each technique in different situations and take note of its effectiveness in reducing stress levels.

4. **Develop a Stress Management Plan:** Develop a personalized stress management plan that incorporates your preferred coping strategies. Create a daily or weekly routine that includes time for stress-relief activities, and prioritize self-care as an essential component of your recovery journey.

5. **Monitor Stress Levels:** Monitor your stress levels regularly and adjust your stress management plan as needed. Stay mindful of your triggers and be proactive in implementing coping strategies to prevent stress from escalating.

Guidance: Identify stressors in your life and brainstorm healthy coping strategies to manage stress effectively.

Experiment with different techniques and develop a personalized stress management plan that supports your sobriety and overall well-being in recovery.

Exploring Lifestyle Changes Worksheet

Description: This worksheet prompts individuals to reflect on lifestyle factors that may contribute to substance use, such as diet, sleep habits, and leisure activities. By identifying areas where positive changes can enhance overall well-being and support recovery goals, individuals can set realistic goals for implementing healthy lifestyle changes.

Time: Set aside 15-20 minutes for this activity.

Activities:

1. **Reflect on Lifestyle Factors:** Reflect on various aspects of your lifestyle, including diet, exercise, sleep habits, leisure activities, and daily routines. Consider how these factors may influence your physical and emotional well-being.
2. **Identify Areas for Improvement:** Identify areas of your lifestyle where positive changes could enhance your overall well-being and support your recovery goals. Consider factors such as nutrition, hydration, exercise, sleep quality, and stress management.
3. **Set Realistic Goals:** Set realistic goals for implementing healthy lifestyle changes based on your reflections. Break down larger goals into

smaller, actionable steps that you can gradually incorporate into your daily routine.

4. **Develop a Plan:** Develop a concrete plan for making and sustaining lifestyle changes. Identify specific actions you can take to improve your diet, exercise routine, sleep hygiene, and leisure activities, and schedule time for these activities in your daily or weekly schedule.

5. **Track Progress:** Track your progress toward your lifestyle goals and make adjustments as needed. Celebrate small victories and stay motivated by focusing on the positive changes you're making to support your recovery journey.

Guidance: Reflect on lifestyle factors that may influence your overall well-being and recovery journey. Identify areas where positive changes can be made and set realistic goals for implementing these changes. Develop a plan for incorporating healthy habits into your daily routine and track your progress over time.

Exploring Social Support Worksheet

Description: This worksheet prompts individuals to assess the level of social support available to them from friends, family, and community resources. By recognizing the importance of social connections in maintaining sobriety and emotional well-being, individuals can cultivate supportive relationships and seek out peer support groups or recovery communities.

Time: Allocate 15-20 minutes for this activity.

Activities:

1. **Assess Social Support:** Reflect on the level of social support available to you from friends, family, and community resources. Consider who you can turn to for emotional support, practical assistance, or encouragement in your recovery journey.

2. **Identify Supportive Relationships:** Identify individuals in your life who provide positive support and encouragement for your sobriety. Consider friends, family members, mentors, therapists, or support group members who understand and respect your recovery goals.

3. **Cultivate Relationships:** Cultivate supportive relationships by investing time and effort in nurturing connections with supportive individuals. Communicate openly about your recovery journey and express gratitude for their support and encouragement.

4. **Seek Out Peer Support:** Seek out peer support groups or recovery communities where you can connect with others who share similar experiences and challenges. Participate in group meetings, online forums, or community events to find support and camaraderie.

5. **Offer Support to Others:** Offer support and encouragement to others who are on their own recovery journeys. By giving back to the community

and helping others, you can strengthen your own sense of purpose and belonging.

Guidance: Assess the level of social support available to you and cultivate supportive relationships that understand and respect your recovery goals. Seek out peer support groups or recovery communities where you can connect with others who share similar experiences and challenges. Use this worksheet as a tool for building a strong support network to aid in your recovery journey.

Exploring Positive Reinforcement Worksheet

Description: This worksheet prompts individuals to reflect on sources of positive reinforcement and rewards that can motivate them to stay sober. By identifying activities, accomplishments, and relationships that bring joy and fulfillment into their lives, individuals can use positive reinforcement to reinforce their commitment to sobriety.

Time: Set aside 15-20 minutes for this activity.

Activities:

1. **Reflect on Sources of Joy:** Reflect on activities, accomplishments, and relationships that bring joy and fulfillment into your life. Consider hobbies, interests, personal achievements, or meaningful connections with others.
2. **Identify Positive Reinforcers:** Identify specific sources of positive reinforcement that can motivate you to stay sober. Consider how these sources of

joy and fulfillment align with your values and support your recovery goals.

3. **Create a Rewards System:** Create a rewards system based on your identified sources of positive reinforcement. Set achievable goals for sobriety milestones or personal achievements and reward yourself with meaningful experiences or treats when you reach these milestones.

4. **Celebrate Successes:** Celebrate your successes and accomplishments along your recovery journey. Acknowledge your progress and the positive changes you're making in your life, and take time to appreciate the moments of joy and fulfillment that come with sobriety.

5. **Stay Motivated:** Use positive reinforcement as a tool for staying motivated and committed to your sobriety. Keep reminders of your sources of joy and fulfillment visible as a source of inspiration and encouragement during challenging times.

Guidance: Reflect on sources of joy and fulfillment in your life and use positive reinforcement to reinforce your commitment to sobriety. Create a rewards system based on achievable goals and celebrate your successes along your recovery journey. Use this worksheet as a tool for staying motivated and focused on your recovery goals.

Exploring Negative Consequences Worksheet

Description: This worksheet prompts individuals to reflect on the negative consequences of substance use, both past and potential future consequences. By considering the physical, emotional, social, and legal repercussions of continued substance abuse, individuals can strengthen their motivation for change.

Time: Allocate 15-20 minutes for this activity.

Activities:

1. **Reflect on Past Consequences:** Reflect on the negative consequences of substance use that you have experienced in the past. Consider how substance abuse has affected your physical health, mental well-being, relationships, and overall quality of life.

2. **Anticipate Future Consequences:** Anticipate potential future consequences of continued substance abuse if you were to relapse. Consider the long-term effects on your health, relationships, finances, career, and legal status.

3. **Evaluate Impact:** Evaluate the impact of negative consequences on your motivation for change. Consider how these consequences have influenced your desire to maintain sobriety and make positive changes in your life.

4. **Strengthen Resolve:** Use your reflections on past and potential future consequences to strengthen

your resolve to stay sober. Remind yourself of the reasons why you decided to pursue recovery and the benefits of living a substance-free life.

5. **Commit to Change:** Commit to making positive changes in your life to avoid or minimize negative consequences associated with substance use. Use your awareness of past consequences as motivation to stay on track with your recovery goals.

Guidance: Reflect on the negative consequences of substance use and use this awareness to strengthen your motivation for change. Consider both past experiences and potential future consequences of continued substance abuse, and commit to making positive changes to support your sobriety and overall well-being.

Exploring Coping Strategies for Cravings Worksheet

Description: This worksheet prompts individuals to identify specific strategies and techniques for managing cravings when they arise. By experimenting with distraction techniques, relaxation exercises, and cognitive-behavioral strategies, individuals can develop a personalized toolkit for managing cravings in different situations.

Time: Set aside 15-20 minutes for this activity.

Activities:

1. **Identify Craving Triggers:** Reflect on situations, emotions, or thoughts that typically trigger cravings for substances. Identify specific triggers that you commonly encounter in your daily life.
2. **Brainstorm Coping Strategies:** Brainstorm a list of coping strategies and techniques that you can use to manage cravings effectively. Consider distraction techniques, relaxation exercises, mindfulness practices, or engaging in enjoyable activities.
3. **Experiment with Techniques:** Experiment with different coping techniques to determine which ones work best for you in managing cravings. Practice using these techniques in various situations to build your skills and confidence in coping with cravings.
4. **Develop a Craving Management Plan:** Develop a personalized craving management plan that incorporates your preferred coping strategies. Create a step-by-step guide for responding to cravings when they arise, and keep this plan handy for quick reference.
5. **Practice Self-Compassion:** Practice self-compassion and patience as you navigate cravings in recovery. Acknowledge the challenges of overcoming cravings and celebrate your efforts in using healthy coping strategies to resist temptation.

Guidance: Identify specific strategies for managing cravings and develop a personalized craving management plan that incorporates your preferred coping techniques.

Practice using these techniques regularly to build your skills and resilience in coping with cravings effectively.

Exploring Self-Care Practices Worksheet

Description: This worksheet prompts individuals to reflect on the importance of self-care in maintaining sobriety and emotional well-being. By identifying self-care activities that nurture physical, emotional, and spiritual health, individuals can prioritize self-care as an essential component of their recovery journey.

Time: Allocate 15-20 minutes for this activity.

Activities:

1. **Reflect on Self-Care Needs:** Reflect on your self-care needs in relation to physical, emotional, and spiritual well-being. Consider activities that nurture each aspect of your health and contribute to overall well-being.
2. **Identify Self-Care Activities:** Identify self-care activities that you enjoy and find rejuvenating. Consider activities such as exercise, meditation, spending time in nature, journaling, creative expression, or connecting with supportive individuals.
3. **Incorporate Self-Care into Daily Routine:** Incorporate self-care activities into your daily or weekly routine. Schedule time for self-care practices and prioritize activities that replenish your energy and nourish your soul.

4. **Practice Mindfulness:** Practice mindfulness and present-moment awareness as you engage in self-care activities. Pay attention to the sensations, thoughts, and emotions that arise during self-care practices, and savor the experience fully.
5. **Prioritize Self-Care:** Prioritize self-care as an essential component of your recovery journey. Recognize that taking care of yourself is not selfish but necessary for maintaining sobriety and emotional well-being.

Guidance: Reflect on the importance of self-care in maintaining sobriety and emotional well-being. Identify self-care activities that nurture physical, emotional, and spiritual health, and prioritize self-care as an essential component of your recovery journey.

Exploring Values and Meaning Worksheet

Description: This worksheet prompts individuals to reflect on their core values, beliefs, and sources of meaning and purpose in life. By connecting with their values and identifying activities and goals that align with their sense of purpose, individuals can use this awareness to guide their decisions and actions in recovery.

Time: Set aside 15-20 minutes for this activity.

Activities:

1. **Reflect on Core Values:** Reflect on your core values and beliefs that guide your life and decision-

making. Consider what matters most to you and what gives your life meaning and purpose.

2. **Identify Meaningful Activities:** Identify activities and goals that align with your core values and sense of purpose. Consider hobbies, interests, relationships, or causes that resonate with your values and contribute to a sense of fulfillment.

3. **Explore Sources of Meaning:** Explore sources of meaning and purpose in your life, both past and present. Reflect on experiences or moments that have brought you a sense of joy, satisfaction, or fulfillment.

4. **Align Actions with Values:** Align your actions and decisions with your core values and sense of purpose. Consider how you can live in accordance with your values in your daily life and recovery journey.

5. **Set Meaningful Goals:** Set meaningful goals that reflect your values and aspirations. Use your awareness of what matters most to you as a guide for setting goals that are aligned with your sense of purpose and contribute to your overall well-being.

Guidance: Reflect on your core values, beliefs, and sources of meaning and purpose in life. Use this awareness to guide your decisions and actions in recovery, and set meaningful goals that align with your values and aspirations.

Reflection on Progress Worksheet

Description: This worksheet prompts individuals to reflect on their progress in substance abuse recovery, including achievements, setbacks, and lessons learned. By celebrating successes, acknowledging challenges, and setting new goals for the future, individuals can reaffirm their commitment to sobriety and continue moving forward in their recovery journey.

Time: Allocate 15-20 minutes for this activity.

Activities:

1. **Celebrate Successes:** Reflect on your achievements and successes in substance abuse recovery. Celebrate milestones, no matter how small, and acknowledge the progress you've made since beginning your recovery journey.
2. **Acknowledge Challenges:** Acknowledge the challenges and obstacles you've faced along the way. Reflect on setbacks or difficult moments, and recognize the strength and resilience you've demonstrated in overcoming adversity.
3. **Identify Lessons Learned:** Identify lessons learned from both successes and challenges in your recovery journey. Consider how these experiences have shaped your growth and contributed to your personal development.
4. **Set New Goals:** Set new goals for your continued recovery journey. Consider areas where you'd like

to focus your efforts and what steps you can take to move closer to your goals.

5. **Reaffirm Commitment:** Reaffirm your commitment to sobriety and overall well-being. Use your reflections on progress as motivation to continue moving forward, one step at a time, in your recovery journey.

Guidance: Reflect on your progress in substance abuse recovery, including achievements, setbacks, and lessons learned. Use this reflection as an opportunity to celebrate successes, acknowledge challenges, and set new goals for the future, reaffirming your commitment to sobriety and overall well-being.

Section 2: Goal Setting and Action Plans

In this section, we focus on setting meaningful goals and creating actionable plans to support substance abuse recovery. Each worksheet provides clear instructions and guidance to help individuals identify their goals, break them down into actionable steps, and stay motivated on their journey towards sobriety.

Identifying Recovery Goals

Description: This worksheet helps individuals identify their overarching recovery goals, including sobriety milestones, personal growth objectives, and lifestyle changes.

Time: Allocate 15-20 minutes for this activity.

Activities:

1. **Reflect on Recovery Goals:** Reflect on your overarching goals for substance abuse recovery. Consider what you hope to achieve in terms of sobriety, personal growth, relationships, health, and overall well-being.
2. **Clarify Objectives:** Clarify specific objectives that align with your recovery goals. Break down larger goals into smaller, manageable steps that you can work towards achieving.
3. **Prioritize Goals:** Prioritize your goals based on their importance and relevance to your recovery journey. Focus on goals that will have the greatest impact on your overall well-being and sobriety.
4. **Write Down Goals:** Write down your recovery goals in a clear and concise manner. Use specific language and measurable criteria to define each goal.
5. **Review and Revise:** Review your goals regularly and revise them as needed based on your progress and evolving priorities in recovery.

Guidance: Reflect on your overarching recovery goals and clarify specific objectives that align with your aspirations. Prioritize your goals and write them down to solidify your commitment to achieving them. Regularly review and revise your goals to stay focused and motivated on your recovery journey.

Creating Action Plans

Description: This worksheet guides individuals in creating actionable plans to achieve their recovery goals. By breaking down goals into concrete steps and identifying potential obstacles, individuals can develop effective strategies for success.

Time: Set aside 20-30 minutes for this activity.

Activities:

1. **Break Down Goals:** Break down each recovery goal into smaller, actionable steps. Consider the specific actions you need to take to make progress towards achieving your goals.
2. **Set Deadlines:** Assign deadlines to each action step to create a sense of urgency and accountability. Be realistic in setting deadlines, taking into account your available time and resources.
3. **Identify Resources:** Identify resources and support systems that can help you achieve your goals. Consider individuals, organizations, or tools that can provide guidance, encouragement, or assistance along the way.

4. **Anticipate Obstacles:** Anticipate potential obstacles or challenges that may arise as you work towards your goals. Develop strategies for overcoming these obstacles and staying on track despite setbacks.

5. **Monitor Progress:** Monitor your progress regularly and track your actions towards each goal. Celebrate small victories and adjust your action plans as needed based on your evolving needs and circumstances.

Guidance: Break down your recovery goals into actionable steps and set deadlines to create momentum and accountability. Identify resources and anticipate obstacles to develop effective strategies for success. Monitor your progress and adjust your action plans as needed to stay on track towards achieving your goals.

Setting Sobriety Milestones

Description: This worksheet helps individuals set sobriety milestones to track their progress and celebrate achievements in recovery.

Time: Allocate 15-20 minutes for this activity.

Activities:

1. **Reflect on Sobriety Goals:** Reflect on your desired level of sobriety and identify milestone markers along your recovery journey. Consider significant timeframes or achievements that represent progress towards your ultimate goal of sobriety.

2. **Define Milestone Markers:** Define specific milestone markers that you will work towards achieving. These markers could include days, weeks, months, or years of sobriety, as well as personal achievements or milestones related to your recovery journey.

3. **Set Rewards:** Associate rewards or incentives with reaching each milestone marker to provide motivation and encouragement. Choose rewards that are meaningful to you and reinforce your commitment to sobriety.

4. **Create a Milestone Tracker:** Create a visual tracker or calendar to monitor your progress towards each sobriety milestone. Mark each milestone as you achieve it and celebrate your accomplishments along the way.

5. **Review and Adjust:** Regularly review your sobriety milestones and adjust them as needed based on your progress and changing circumstances in recovery.

Guidance: Set sobriety milestones to track your progress and celebrate achievements in recovery. Define specific markers, associate rewards with reaching milestones, and create a visual tracker to monitor your progress. Regularly review and adjust your milestones to stay motivated and focused on your journey towards sobriety.

Developing Daily Habits

Description: This worksheet helps individuals identify daily habits and routines that support their recovery goals and promote sobriety.

Time: Set aside 15-20 minutes for this activity.

Activities:

1. **Reflect on Daily Routines:** Reflect on your current daily habits and routines, considering how they support or hinder your recovery goals. Identify habits that contribute to your overall well-being and sobriety, as well as those that may be detrimental to your progress.

2. **Set Positive Habits:** Identify positive habits and routines that you would like to incorporate into your daily life to support your recovery. These could include habits related to self-care, stress management, healthy coping strategies, and sobriety maintenance.

3. **Create a Daily Schedule:** Create a daily schedule or routine that incorporates your desired habits and activities. Allocate time for self-care, exercise, relaxation, hobbies, and other activities that promote your overall well-being and support your recovery goals.

4. **Track Progress:** Track your adherence to your daily habits and routines using a journal or habit tracker.

Monitor your consistency and identify areas for improvement or adjustment as needed.

5. **Adjust as Needed:** Regularly review your daily habits and routines and adjust them as needed based on your progress and evolving needs in recovery. Be flexible and open to making changes that better support your sobriety and overall well-being.

Guidance: Identify daily habits and routines that support your recovery goals and promote sobriety. Create a daily schedule that incorporates positive habits related to self-care, stress management, and sobriety maintenance. Track your progress and adjust your habits as needed to support your ongoing recovery journey.

Establishing Healthy Boundaries

Description: This worksheet guides individuals in establishing healthy boundaries to protect their sobriety and well-being in relationships and interactions with others.

Time: Allocate 20-30 minutes for this activity.

Activities:

1. **Reflect on Relationship Dynamics:** Reflect on your current relationships and interactions with others, considering how they impact your sobriety and overall well-being. Identify relationships or

situations where boundaries may be needed to protect your recovery.

2. **Identify Boundary Needs:** Identify specific boundaries that you need to establish in order to protect your sobriety and well-being. Consider boundaries related to substance use, communication, time management, and personal space.

3. **Communicate Boundaries:** Communicate your boundaries assertively and clearly to others involved. Use "I" statements to express your needs and expectations, and be firm in enforcing your boundaries.

4. **Set Consequences:** Set consequences for boundary violations and communicate them to others involved. Establish clear consequences that are appropriate to the situation and enforce them consistently.

5. **Practice Self-Care:** Prioritize self-care and emotional well-being as you navigate boundary-setting in relationships. Practice self-compassion and seek support from others as needed to maintain your boundaries and protect your recovery.

Guidance: Reflect on your relationship dynamics and identify boundaries needed to protect your sobriety and well-being. Communicate boundaries assertively, set consequences for boundary violations, and prioritize self-care as you navigate boundary-setting in relationships

Building Support Networks

Description: This worksheet helps individuals identify and cultivate supportive relationships and networks to bolster their recovery journey.

Time: Allocate 20-30 minutes for this activity.

Activities:

1. **Identify Supportive Individuals:** Reflect on your existing support network and identify individuals who offer encouragement, understanding, and assistance in your recovery journey.
2. **Expand Support Network:** Identify potential sources of support outside your current network, such as support groups, recovery communities, mentors, or therapists.
3. **Reach Out:** Take proactive steps to reach out to individuals or groups who can provide support and encouragement. Attend support group meetings, reach out to peers in recovery, or seek guidance from a mentor or therapist.
4. **Nurture Relationships:** Invest time and effort in nurturing supportive relationships and connections. Be open and honest about your recovery journey and express gratitude for the support you receive.
5. **Offer Support:** Be willing to offer support to others in recovery as well. Share your experiences, offer encouragement, and be a source of inspiration to those who may be struggling.

Guidance: Build a strong support network by identifying supportive individuals and reaching out to potential sources of support outside your current network. Nurture relationships with supportive individuals and offer support

Setting Health and Wellness Goals

Description: This worksheet guides individuals in setting health and wellness goals that promote physical, emotional, and mental well-being in recovery.

Time: Set aside 15-20 minutes for this activity.

Activities:

1. **Reflect on Health Priorities:** Reflect on your current health status and identify areas where you would like to make improvements. Consider physical, emotional, and mental aspects of health.
2. **Set Specific Goals:** Set specific, measurable goals related to improving your health and wellness. These could include goals related to exercise, nutrition, sleep, stress management, or mental health.
3. **Break Down Goals:** Break down larger health goals into smaller, actionable steps that you can work towards achieving. Consider what specific actions you need to take to make progress towards each goal.
4. **Create a Wellness Plan:** Create a wellness plan that outlines your health and wellness goals, as well as the actions you will take to achieve them. Include

deadlines and accountability measures to stay on track.

5. **Monitor Progress:** Monitor your progress towards your health and wellness goals regularly. Track your actions and achievements, and celebrate milestones along the way.

Guidance: Set specific health and wellness goals that promote physical, emotional, and mental well-being in recovery. Break down goals into actionable steps, create a wellness plan, and monitor your progress regularly to stay on track towards achieving your health goals.

Financial Planning for Recovery

Description: This worksheet helps individuals assess their financial situation and create a plan for managing finances in recovery.

Time: Allocate 20-30 minutes for this activity.

Activities:

1. **Assess Financial Situation:** Assess your current financial situation, including income, expenses, debts, and savings. Identify areas where you may need to make changes or adjustments to support your recovery goals.

2. **Set Financial Goals:** Set specific financial goals related to managing debts, building savings, reducing expenses, or increasing income. Consider both short-term and long-term financial objectives.

3. **Create a Budget:** Create a budget that outlines your income and expenses, as well as your financial goals. Allocate funds towards essentials such as housing, food, and healthcare, as well as towards savings and debt repayment.
4. **Track Spending:** Track your spending regularly to ensure that you are staying within your budget and making progress towards your financial goals. Use tools such as budgeting apps or spreadsheets to track your expenses.
5. **Seek Financial Support:** Seek support from financial professionals or support groups if you need assistance with managing your finances. Consider reaching out to a financial advisor, counselor, or support group for guidance and advice.

Guidance: Assess your financial situation and set specific goals for managing finances in recovery. Create a budget, track your spending, and seek support from financial professionals or support groups as needed to achieve your financial goals.

Developing Career and Educational Goals

Description: This worksheet guides individuals in setting career and educational goals to support their long-term recovery and personal growth.

Time: Set aside 20-30 minutes for this activity.

Activities:

1. **Reflect on Career Aspirations:** Reflect on your career aspirations and educational goals, considering how they align with your recovery journey and overall well-being.
2. **Identify Career Paths:** Identify potential career paths or educational opportunities that interest you and align with your skills, interests, and values.
3. **Set Specific Goals:** Set specific, measurable goals related to advancing your career or education. These could include goals related to acquiring new skills, obtaining certifications, or pursuing higher education.
4. **Create an Action Plan:** Create an action plan that outlines the steps you need to take to achieve your career and educational goals. Break down larger goals into smaller, actionable steps and set deadlines for each step.
5. **Seek Support and Resources:** Seek support and resources to help you achieve your career and educational goals. Consider reaching out to career counselors, educational institutions, or professional organizations for guidance and assistance.

Guidance: Set specific career and educational goals that support your long-term recovery and personal growth. Create an action plan, seek support and resources, and take proactive steps towards achieving your goals in career and education.

Improving Relationships and Communication Skills

Description: This worksheet helps individuals identify areas for improvement in their relationships and communication skills, and set goals for enhancing interpersonal interactions in recovery.

Time: Allocate 20-30 minutes for this activity.

Activities:

1. **Reflect on Relationship Dynamics:** Reflect on your current relationships and communication patterns, considering areas where improvement is needed. Identify common challenges or conflicts in your relationships.

2. **Identify Communication Goals:** Identify specific communication goals that you would like to work towards achieving in your relationships. These could include goals related to active listening, expressing emotions, setting boundaries, or resolving conflicts.

3. **Practice Empathy:** Practice empathy and understanding in your interactions with others. Put yourself in the shoes of the other person and try to see things from their perspective.

4. **Develop Assertiveness:** Develop assertiveness skills to express your needs, opinions, and boundaries clearly and respectfully. Practice assertive

communication techniques such as using "I" statements and setting boundaries.

5. **Seek Feedback:** Seek feedback from trusted individuals or professionals on your communication skills and interpersonal interactions. Use constructive feedback to identify areas for improvement and adjust your approach accordingly.

Guidance: Identify areas for improvement in your relationships and communication skills, and set specific goals for enhancing interpersonal interactions in recovery. Practice empathy, develop assertiveness, and seek feedback to improve your communication skills and relationships.

Cultivating Healthy Habits

Description: This worksheet assists individuals in cultivating healthy habits that support their overall well-being and promote long-term recovery.

Time: Allocate 15-20 minutes for this activity.

Activities:

1. **Reflect on Current Habits:** Reflect on your current habits and routines, considering their impact on your physical, mental, and emotional health. Identify habits that contribute to your well-being as well as those that may be detrimental to your recovery.

2. **Identify Healthy Habits:** Identify healthy habits that you would like to cultivate to support your recovery journey. These could include habits related to nutrition, exercise, sleep, mindfulness, and self-care.

3. **Set SMART Goals:** Set SMART (Specific, Measurable, Achievable, Relevant, Time-bound) goals for cultivating healthy habits. Define each goal clearly and establish criteria for measuring your progress.

4. **Create a Habit Tracker:** Create a habit tracker to monitor your adherence to healthy habits on a daily or weekly basis. Use the tracker to record your actions and track your progress over time.

5. **Celebrate Progress:** Celebrate your progress and achievements as you cultivate healthy habits. Acknowledge your efforts and successes, no matter how small, and use positive reinforcement to stay motivated.

Guidance: Reflect on your current habits and identify healthy habits to cultivate in support of your recovery journey. Set SMART goals, create a habit tracker, and celebrate your progress as you develop and maintain healthy habits.

Enhancing Self-Esteem and Self-Confidence

Description: This worksheet helps individuals enhance their self-esteem and self-confidence, which are essential for maintaining sobriety and achieving personal growth in recovery.

Time: Set aside 20-30 minutes for this activity.

Activities:

1. **Identify Strengths:** Identify your strengths, talents, and positive qualities. Reflect on past achievements and successes, no matter how small, to boost your confidence.
2. **Challenge Negative Beliefs:** Challenge negative beliefs and self-doubt that may undermine your self-esteem. Replace negative thoughts with positive affirmations and realistic self-appraisals.
3. **Set Achievable Goals:** Set achievable goals that align with your strengths and values. Break down larger goals into smaller, manageable steps, and celebrate each accomplishment along the way.
4. **Practice Self-Compassion:** Practice self-compassion and kindness towards yourself, especially during challenging times. Treat yourself with the same care and understanding that you would offer to a close friend.
5. **Seek Support:** Seek support from others who can offer encouragement and validation. Surround

yourself with positive influences and avoid negative influences that may erode your self-esteem.

Guidance: Enhance your self-esteem and self-confidence by identifying your strengths, challenging negative beliefs, and setting achievable goals. Practice self-compassion and seek support from others to cultivate a positive self-image in recovery.

Assertiveness Training

Description: This worksheet provides training in assertiveness skills, empowering individuals to communicate their needs, express their opinions, and set boundaries effectively.

Time: Allocate 20-30 minutes for this activity.

Activities:

1. **Understand Assertiveness:** Understand the concept of assertiveness and its importance in interpersonal communication. Recognize the difference between assertive, aggressive, and passive communication styles.
2. **Identify Assertive Behaviors:** Identify assertive behaviors, such as using "I" statements, expressing feelings and opinions honestly, and standing up for your rights without violating the rights of others.
3. **Practice Assertive Communication:** Practice assertive communication skills in various scenarios,

such as expressing preferences, setting boundaries, and refusing requests politely but firmly.

4. **Role-Playing Exercises:** Engage in role-playing exercises with a partner or therapist to practice assertive communication in realistic situations. Receive feedback on your communication style and adjust as needed.

5. **Apply Assertiveness Skills:** Apply assertiveness skills in your daily interactions and relationships. Start with low-risk situations and gradually work up to more challenging scenarios as you build confidence in your communication abilities.

Guidance: Learn and practice assertiveness skills to communicate effectively, express your needs, and set boundaries in recovery. Use role-playing exercises and real-life scenarios to develop and apply assertive communication skills in various situations.

Overcoming Procrastination

Description: This worksheet helps individuals overcome procrastination, a common barrier to progress and success in recovery, by identifying underlying causes and implementing effective strategies.

Time: Set aside 20-30 minutes for this activity.

Activities:

1. **Understand Procrastination:** Understand the underlying causes and consequences of

procrastination. Recognize common triggers and patterns that contribute to procrastination in your life.

2. **Identify Procrastination Patterns:** Identify specific tasks or responsibilities that you tend to procrastinate on. Consider the reasons why you avoid these tasks, such as fear of failure, perfectionism, or lack of motivation.

3. **Break Tasks Down:** Break down larger tasks into smaller, more manageable steps. Set clear deadlines and establish a timeline for completing each step to create a sense of urgency and accountability.

4. **Eliminate Distractions:** Identify and eliminate distractions that contribute to procrastination, such as social media, television, or disorganized workspaces. Create a conducive environment for productivity and focus.

5. **Reward Progress:** Reward yourself for making progress and meeting deadlines, no matter how small. Use positive reinforcement to motivate yourself and reinforce productive behaviors.

Guidance: Overcome procrastination by understanding its causes, identifying procrastination patterns, and implementing strategies to increase productivity and focus. Break tasks down, eliminate distractions, and reward progress to overcome procrastination effectively.

Time Management Skills

Description: This worksheet provides training in time management skills, helping individuals prioritize tasks, set goals, and use time effectively to support their recovery journey.

Time: Allocate 20-30 minutes for this activity.

Activities:

1. **Set Clear Goals:** Set clear and specific goals for your recovery journey and other areas of your life. Break down larger goals into smaller, actionable steps, and establish deadlines for each step.
2. **Prioritize Tasks:** Prioritize tasks based on their importance and urgency. Use techniques such as the Eisenhower Matrix or ABC prioritization to categorize tasks and focus on high-priority activities.
3. **Create a Schedule:** Create a daily or weekly schedule that allocates time for essential activities, including self-care, work or school, recovery meetings, and leisure activities. Use digital or paper planners to organize your schedule effectively.
4. **Manage Distractions:** Identify and minimize distractions that may interfere with your productivity and focus. Set boundaries with technology, create designated workspaces, and use time-blocking techniques to maintain focus.

5. **Review and Adjust:** Regularly review your schedule and task list to ensure that you are staying on track towards your goals. Adjust your schedule and priorities as needed based on changes in your circumstances or priorities.

Guidance: Develop effective time management skills by setting clear goals, prioritizing tasks, creating a schedule, managing distractions, and reviewing your progress regularly. Use time management techniques to maximize productivity and support your recovery journey.

Stress Management Techniques

Description: This worksheet explores various stress management techniques and helps individuals develop a personalized toolkit for coping with stress in recovery.

Time: Set aside 20-30 minutes for this activity.

Activities:

1. **Identify Stressors:** Identify sources of stress in your life, both internal and external. Reflect on situations, events, or thoughts that trigger stress reactions and contribute to emotional distress.
2. **Explore Coping Techniques:** Explore a variety of stress management techniques, including relaxation exercises, mindfulness practices, deep breathing exercises, and physical activities such as exercise or yoga.

3. **Experiment with Techniques:** Experiment with different stress management techniques to determine which ones work best for you. Pay attention to how each technique affects your mood, stress levels, and overall well-being.
4. **Create a Stress Management Plan:** Create a personalized stress management plan that outlines the techniques you will use to cope with stress in different situations. Include specific strategies for managing acute stressors and preventing chronic stress.
5. **Practice Self-Care:** Prioritize self-care activities that promote relaxation, self-soothing, and emotional well-being. Incorporate regular self-care practices into your daily routine to reduce stress and support your recovery journey.

Guidance: Develop a personalized toolkit for coping with stress in recovery by identifying stressors, exploring coping techniques, and creating a stress management plan. Practice self-care and incorporate stress management techniques into your daily routine to promote emotional well-being.

Developing Problem-Solving Skills

Description: This worksheet helps individuals develop problem-solving skills to effectively address challenges and obstacles encountered in recovery.

Time: Allocate 20-30 minutes for this activity.

Activities:

1. **Understand Problem-Solving Process:** Understand the problem-solving process, which involves identifying problems, generating potential solutions, evaluating alternatives, and implementing effective solutions.
2. **Identify Challenges:** Identify specific challenges or obstacles that you are currently facing in your recovery journey. Consider both internal and external factors that may be contributing to these challenges.
3. **Generate Solutions:** Brainstorm potential solutions to each identified challenge, without censoring or evaluating ideas at this stage. Be creative and open-minded in generating alternative solutions.
4. **Evaluate Options:** Evaluate the pros and cons of each potential solution, considering factors such as feasibility, effectiveness, and potential consequences. Select the most promising solution based on your assessment.
5. **Implement Solutions:** Implement the chosen solution and take proactive steps to address the identified challenge. Monitor the outcomes of your actions and be prepared to adjust your approach if necessary.

Guidance: Develop problem-solving skills by understanding the problem-solving process, identifying challenges, generating solutions, evaluating options, and implementing effective solutions in recovery.

Building Resilience

Description: This worksheet explores resilience, the ability to bounce back from adversity, and helps individuals develop resilience-building strategies to navigate challenges in recovery.

Time: Set aside 20-30 minutes for this activity.

Activities:

1. **Understand Resilience:** Understand the concept of resilience and its importance in recovery. Recognize that resilience is a skill that can be developed through practice and self-awareness.
2. **Identify Resilience Factors:** Identify factors that contribute to resilience, such as social support, problem-solving skills, optimism, and self-efficacy. Reflect on your own strengths and resources that can help you bounce back from adversity.
3. **Cultivate Positive Thinking:** Cultivate a positive outlook and practice optimism in the face of challenges. Focus on solutions rather than dwelling on problems, and challenge negative thinking patterns that undermine resilience.
4. **Seek Support:** Seek support from others who can provide encouragement, guidance, and perspective during difficult times. Build a strong support

network of friends, family, peers, and professionals who can offer assistance.

5. **Practice Self-Care:** Prioritize self-care activities that nurture your physical, emotional, and mental well-being. Engage in activities that promote relaxation, stress reduction, and emotional regulation to enhance resilience.

Guidance: Develop resilience-building strategies by understanding resilience, identifying resilience factors, cultivating positive thinking, seeking support, and prioritizing self-care activities in recovery.

Improving Decision-Making Skills

Description: This worksheet helps individuals improve their decision-making skills, enabling them to make informed and effective choices in recovery.

Time: Allocate 20-30 minutes for this activity.

Activities:

1. **Understand Decision-Making Process:** Understand the decision-making process, which involves identifying options, gathering information, evaluating alternatives, and making a choice based on rational assessment.
2. **Clarify Goals:** Clarify your goals and priorities in recovery, considering both short-term and long-term objectives. Align your decisions with your values, aspirations, and desired outcomes.

3. **Gather Information:** Gather relevant information and facts to inform your decision-making process. Consider various perspectives, seek advice from trusted sources, and weigh the potential consequences of each option.
4. **Evaluate Alternatives:** Evaluate the pros and cons of each alternative, considering factors such as feasibility, desirability, and potential risks. Use decision-making tools such as decision matrices or cost-benefit analyses to facilitate evaluation.
5. **Make a Decision:** Make a decision based on your assessment of the available options and the information gathered. Trust your judgment and be prepared to take responsibility for the consequences of your decision.

Guidance: Improve decision-making skills by understanding the decision-making process, clarifying goals, gathering information, evaluating alternatives, and making informed choices in recovery.

Setting Boundaries with Substances

Description: This worksheet helps individuals set and maintain boundaries with substances to protect their sobriety and well-being in recovery.

Time: Set aside 20-30 minutes for this activity.

Activities:

1. **Understand Boundary Setting:** Understand the concept of boundary setting and its importance in recovery. Recognize that setting boundaries with substances involves defining limits and rules to protect your sobriety and well-being.
2. **Identify Triggers:** Identify triggers and situations that may tempt you to use substances, such as social gatherings, stress, or emotional distress. Recognize the warning signs of potential relapse and take proactive steps to address them.
3. **Establish Clear Rules:** Establish clear and specific rules regarding substance use, including abstinence goals, limits on exposure to triggering environments, and guidelines for managing cravings or urges.
4. **Communicate Boundaries:** Communicate your boundaries assertively and clearly to others involved. Use "I" statements to express your needs and expectations, and be firm in enforcing your boundaries.
5. **Set Consequences:** Set consequences for boundary violations and communicate them to others involved. Establish clear consequences that are appropriate to the situation and enforce them consistently.
6. **Practice Self-Care:** Prioritize self-care and emotional well-being as you navigate boundary-setting in relationships. Practice self-compassion and seek support from others as needed to

maintain your boundaries and protect your recovery.

Guidance: Reflect on your relationship dynamics and identify boundaries needed to protect your sobriety and well-being. Communicate boundaries assertively, set consequences for boundary violations, and prioritize self-care as you navigate boundary-setting in relationships.

Developing Healthy Relationships

Description: This worksheet assists individuals in developing healthy relationships that support their recovery journey and contribute to their overall well-being.

Time: Allocate 20-30 minutes for this activity.

Activities:

1. **Reflect on Relationship Patterns:** Reflect on past relationship patterns and dynamics, considering how they may have influenced your substance use and recovery journey. Identify unhealthy patterns to avoid and healthy qualities to cultivate in relationships.
2. **Clarify Relationship Values:** Clarify your values and priorities in relationships, considering what qualities you seek in healthy connections. Align your relationship values with your recovery goals and personal aspirations.
3. **Set Boundaries:** Set clear and appropriate boundaries in relationships to protect your sobriety

and well-being. Communicate your boundaries assertively and enforce them consistently to maintain healthy boundaries.

4. **Seek Supportive Connections:** Seek out supportive connections and relationships that align with your values and support your recovery journey. Surround yourself with individuals who encourage your growth and well-being.

5. **Practice Effective Communication:** Practice effective communication skills in relationships, including active listening, assertive expression of needs, and empathy. Foster open and honest communication to build trust and understanding.

6. **Cultivate Empathy and Compassion:** Cultivate empathy and compassion in your interactions with others, recognizing their perspectives and experiences. Practice empathy and compassion towards yourself as well, embracing self-acceptance and understanding.

7. **Resolve Conflict Constructively:** Learn to resolve conflicts and disagreements constructively in relationships, focusing on finding mutually beneficial solutions and maintaining respect and empathy for each other.

8. **Prioritize Self-Care:** Prioritize self-care and emotional well-being as you navigate relationships in recovery. Take time for self-reflection, relaxation, and activities that nurture your overall health and happiness.

Guidance: Develop healthy relationships by reflecting on past patterns, clarifying relationship values, setting boundaries, seeking supportive connections, practicing effective communication, cultivating empathy and compassion, resolving conflict constructively, and prioritizing self-care.

Building Social Support Networks

Description: This worksheet helps individuals build and strengthen their social support networks, which are essential for maintaining sobriety and emotional well-being in recovery.

Time: Set aside 20-30 minutes for this activity.

Activities:

1. **Understand Social Support:** Understand the importance of social support in recovery, including emotional support, practical assistance, and encouragement from others.
2. **Identify Supportive Individuals:** Identify individuals in your life who offer support and encouragement for your recovery journey. Consider family members, friends, peers, mentors, therapists, and support group members.
3. **Assess Relationships:** Assess the quality and depth of your current relationships, considering the level of support and understanding they provide. Identify relationships that are supportive and

nurturing, as well as those that may be detrimental to your recovery.

4. **Expand Support Network:** Expand your support network by reaching out to new connections and resources. Consider joining support groups, attending recovery meetings, volunteering in your community, or participating in social activities that align with your interests.

5. **Communicate Needs:** Communicate your needs and preferences to supportive individuals in your network. Be open and honest about your recovery journey, and express gratitude for their support and encouragement.

6. **Offer Support to Others:** Offer support and encouragement to others in your social support network. Build reciprocal relationships based on mutual understanding, empathy, and respect.

7. **Maintain Connections:** Maintain regular contact with supportive individuals in your network, even during times of stability. Cultivate meaningful connections and nurture relationships that contribute positively to your recovery and well-being.

Guidance: Build and strengthen your social support network by identifying supportive individuals, assessing relationships, expanding your network, communicating your needs, offering support to others, and maintaining regular contact with supportive connections.

Enhancing Interpersonal Skills

Description: This worksheet helps individuals enhance their interpersonal skills, including communication, empathy, active listening, and conflict resolution, to improve their relationships and social interactions in recovery.

Time: Allocate 20-30 minutes for this activity.

Activities:

1. **Understand Interpersonal Skills:** Understand the importance of interpersonal skills in building and maintaining healthy relationships. Recognize the impact of effective communication, empathy, active listening, and conflict resolution on relationship dynamics.

2. **Assess Interpersonal Strengths and Weaknesses:** Assess your current interpersonal skills, identifying strengths and areas for improvement. Reflect on past interactions and relationships to gain insight into your communication style and relational patterns.

3. **Set Interpersonal Goals:** Set specific and achievable goals for enhancing your interpersonal skills in recovery. Focus on areas such as assertive communication, empathetic listening, and constructive conflict resolution.

4. **Practice Active Listening:** Practice active listening skills in your interactions with others, focusing on understanding their perspectives, feelings, and needs. Avoid interrupting, judging, or dismissing the speaker's thoughts or emotions.

5. **Express Empathy and Understanding:** Express empathy and understanding towards others, acknowledging their experiences and validating their feelings. Practice empathy by putting yourself in their shoes and responding with compassion.

6. **Communicate Assertively:** Practice assertive communication skills in your interactions, expressing your thoughts, feelings, and needs openly and respectfully. Use "I" statements to convey your messages and set clear boundaries when necessary.

7. **Resolve Conflict Constructively:** Learn to resolve conflicts and disagreements constructively in your relationships. Focus on finding mutually beneficial solutions and maintaining respect and understanding for each other's perspectives.

8. **Seek Feedback:** Seek feedback from trusted individuals in your network on your interpersonal skills and communication style. Be open to constructive criticism and use it as an opportunity for growth and self-improvement.

Guidance: Enhance your interpersonal skills by understanding their importance, assessing strengths and weaknesses, setting goals, practicing active listening, expressing empathy, communicating assertively, resolving conflict constructively, and seeking feedback for improvement.

Assertive Communication in Relationships

Description: This worksheet focuses specifically on assertive communication skills within relationships, empowering individuals to express their needs, feelings, and boundaries effectively.

Time: Set aside 20-30 minutes for this activity.

Activities:

1. **Understand Assertive Communication:** Understand the concept of assertive communication and its role in healthy relationships. Recognize the benefits of assertive communication, including improved clarity, honesty, and mutual respect.
2. **Identify Communication Styles:** Identify different communication styles, including passive, aggressive, and passive-aggressive, and their respective characteristics. Reflect on your own communication style and its impact on your relationships.
3. **Practice Assertive Expression:** Practice assertive expression of thoughts, feelings, and needs in various relationship scenarios. Use "I" statements to convey your messages assertively and respectfully, without blaming or criticizing others.

4. **Set and Enforce Boundaries:** Set clear and appropriate boundaries in your relationships, communicating them assertively and consistently. Be firm in enforcing your boundaries and assertive in responding to boundary violations.
5. **Handle Criticism and Feedback:** Handle criticism and feedback from others assertively and constructively. Listen attentively to the feedback, acknowledge valid points, and express your thoughts and feelings assertively in response.
6. **Negotiate Compromises:** Practice negotiating compromises and solutions in your relationships, focusing on finding win-win outcomes that satisfy the needs and interests of all parties involved.
7. **Seek Support:** Seek support and encouragement from others as you practice assertive communication skills. Surround yourself with individuals who respect your assertiveness and provide positive reinforcement for your efforts.
8. **Reflect on Progress:** Reflect on your progress in developing assertive communication skills, celebrating successes and identifying areas for further growth. Recognize that assertiveness is a skill that improves with practice and self-awareness.

Guidance: Develop assertive communication skills by understanding its importance, identifying communication styles, practicing assertive expression, setting and enforcing boundaries, handling criticism and feedback, negotiating compromises, seeking support, and reflecting on progress.

Improving Conflict Resolution Skills

Description: This worksheet helps individuals improve their conflict resolution skills, enabling them to address disagreements and conflicts constructively in their relationships.

Time: Allocate 20-30 minutes for this activity.

Activities:

1. **Understand Conflict Resolution:** Understand the concept of conflict resolution and its importance in maintaining healthy relationships. Recognize that conflicts are a natural part of relationships and provide opportunities for growth and understanding.
2. **Identify Conflict Styles:** Identify different conflict resolution styles, including avoidance, accommodation, competition, compromise, and collaboration. Reflect on your preferred conflict style and its effectiveness in resolving conflicts.
3. **Practice Active Listening:** Practice active listening skills in conflict situations, focusing on understanding the perspectives and feelings of all parties involved. Listen attentively without interrupting or judging, and paraphrase to ensure understanding.

4. **Express Thoughts and Feelings:** Express your thoughts and feelings assertively and respectfully during conflicts, using "I" statements to convey your perspective. Avoid blaming or criticizing others and focus on expressing your own needs and concerns.

5. **Seek Common Ground:** Seek common ground and areas of agreement with the other party, focusing on shared goals and interests. Look for win-win solutions that address the needs and concerns of both parties involved.

6. **Brainstorm Solutions:** Brainstorm potential solutions to the conflict, considering a range of options and alternatives. Be creative and open-minded in generating ideas, and evaluate each solution based on its feasibility and effectiveness.

7. **Negotiate Compromises:** Negotiate compromises and agreements that satisfy the needs and interests of all parties involved. Be willing to make concessions and seek mutually acceptable solutions to the conflict.

8. **Follow Up and Reflect:** Follow up on the resolution of the conflict and reflect on the outcome. Identify lessons learned from the conflict resolution process and apply them to future interactions and conflicts.

Guidance: Improve conflict resolution skills by understanding its importance, identifying conflict styles, practicing active listening, expressing thoughts and feelings assertively, seeking common ground, brainstorming solutions, negotiating compromises, following up, and reflecting on outcomes.

Developing Empathy and Understanding

Description: This worksheet focuses on developing empathy and understanding in relationships, fostering deeper connections and mutual respect with others.

Time: Set aside 20-30 minutes for this activity.

Activities:

1. **Understand Empathy:** Understand the concept of empathy and its importance in building strong and meaningful relationships. Recognize empathy as the ability to understand and share the feelings of others.
2. **Practice Perspective-Taking:** Practice perspective-taking skills by putting yourself in the shoes of others and seeing the world from their point of view. Imagine their thoughts, feelings, and experiences to cultivate empathy and understanding.
3. **Listen Actively:** Listen actively to others, paying attention to their words, tone, and body language. Show genuine interest and empathy in their experiences, and validate their feelings and emotions.
4. **Express Empathy:** Express empathy and understanding towards others in your interactions.

Acknowledge their feelings and experiences, and respond with compassion and support.

5. **Validate Emotions:** Validate the emotions of others by acknowledging their feelings and experiences as valid and understandable. Avoid judgment or criticism and focus on creating a safe and supportive space for emotional expression.

6. **Show Empathy Through Actions:** Show empathy through your actions and behaviors, demonstrating care, compassion, and support for others in need. Offer practical assistance or emotional support as appropriate to show that you understand and care about their well-being.

7. **Practice Self-Compassion:** Practice self-compassion and understanding towards yourself, acknowledging your own feelings and experiences with kindness and acceptance. Treat yourself with the same empathy and understanding that you extend to others.

8. **Reflect on Interactions:** Reflect on your interactions with others, considering the level of empathy and understanding you demonstrate. Identify opportunities for improvement and commit to practicing empathy and understanding in your relationships.

Guidance: Develop empathy and understanding in relationships by understanding its importance, practicing perspective-taking, listening actively, expressing empathy, validating emotions, showing empathy through actions, practicing self-compassion, and reflecting on interactions.

Navigating Peer Pressure

Description: This worksheet helps individuals navigate peer pressure and influence, empowering them to make confident and independent choices in their recovery journey.

Time: Allocate 20-30 minutes for this activity.

Activities:

1. **Understand Peer Pressure:** Understand the concept of peer pressure and its influence on behavior, thoughts, and decisions. Recognize that peer pressure can be both positive and negative, and learn to distinguish between the two.
2. **Identify Sources of Peer Pressure:** Identify sources of peer pressure in your life, including friends, family, social groups, and cultural norms. Recognize situations where peer pressure may arise and the potential impact on your recovery journey.
3. **Assess Personal Values:** Assess your personal values, beliefs, and priorities, considering how they align with or differ from the expectations of others. Clarify your boundaries and commitments in relation to substance use and recovery.
4. **Practice Assertiveness:** Practice assertiveness skills in dealing with peer pressure, asserting your own thoughts, feelings, and decisions confidently and

respectfully. Learn to say no assertively and set boundaries with others.

5. **Seek Supportive Connections:** Seek out supportive connections and relationships that respect and support your recovery goals. Surround yourself with individuals who encourage your growth and well-being and respect your decisions.

6. **Cultivate Confidence:** Cultivate confidence in your ability to make independent choices and resist negative peer influence. Trust your judgment and intuition, and believe in your capacity to stay true to your values and commitments.

7. **Develop Coping Strategies:** Develop coping strategies to deal with peer pressure effectively, such as practicing refusal skills, finding alternative social activities, and seeking support from trusted individuals.

8. **Reflect on Peer Influence:** Reflect on the influence of peers and social groups in your life, considering how they shape your behavior and decisions. Identify positive influences that support your recovery and negative influences that may hinder your progress.

Guidance: Navigate peer pressure by understanding its influence, identifying sources of pressure, assessing personal values, practicing assertiveness, seeking supportive connections, cultivating confidence, developing coping strategies, and reflecting on peer influence.

Building Trust in Relationships

Description: This worksheet focuses on building trust in relationships, fostering a sense of safety, reliability, and mutual respect with others.

Time: Set aside 20-30 minutes for this activity.

Activities:

1. **Understand Trust:** Understand the concept of trust and its importance in building healthy and meaningful relationships. Recognize trust as the foundation of strong connections based on reliability, honesty, and integrity.
2. **Reflect on Trust:** Reflect on your experiences with trust in past relationships, considering times when trust was present or broken. Identify factors that contribute to trust-building and trust erosion in relationships.
3. **Assess Trustworthiness:** Assess your own trustworthiness in relationships, considering how your words, actions, and behaviors influence others' trust in you. Identify areas where you can improve trust-building behaviors and qualities.
4. **Communicate Openly:** Communicate openly and honestly in your relationships, sharing your thoughts, feelings, and intentions authentically. Be transparent about your actions and decisions to build trust with others.

5. **Demonstrate Reliability:** Demonstrate reliability and consistency in your actions and commitments, following through on promises and agreements. Show that you can be counted on to fulfill your responsibilities and obligations.

6. **Practice Vulnerability:** Practice vulnerability in relationships by sharing your fears, insecurities, and vulnerabilities with trusted individuals. Be willing to be open and authentic, even if it involves some level of risk.

7. **Show Empathy and Understanding:** Show empathy and understanding towards others' experiences and emotions, validating their feelings and perspectives. Demonstrate empathy as a way of building connection and trust with others.

8. **Repair Trust When Broken:** Learn to repair trust in relationships when it is broken, acknowledging mistakes or breaches of trust and taking steps to rebuild it. Apologize sincerely, make amends, and demonstrate changed behavior over time.

Guidance: Build trust in relationships by understanding its importance, reflecting on trust experiences, assessing trustworthiness, communicating openly, demonstrating reliability, practicing vulnerability, showing empathy and understanding, and repairing trust when broken.

Setting Healthy Boundaries

Description: This worksheet assists individuals in setting healthy boundaries in relationships, empowering them to protect their well-being and maintain autonomy.

Time: Allocate 20-30 minutes for this activity.

Activities:

1. **Understand Boundaries:** Understand the concept of boundaries and their importance in relationships. Recognize that boundaries define the limits and expectations of acceptable behavior in relationships.
2. **Reflect on Boundary Violations:** Reflect on past experiences of boundary violations in relationships, considering how they affected your well-being and autonomy. Identify situations where boundaries were crossed or disregarded.
3. **Clarify Personal Boundaries:** Clarify your personal boundaries and limits in various areas of your life, including physical, emotional, and social boundaries. Identify behaviors or actions that are acceptable or unacceptable to you.
4. **Communicate Boundaries Assertively:** Communicate your boundaries assertively and respectfully to others, expressing your needs, preferences, and limits clearly and directly. Use "I" statements to convey your boundaries without blaming or criticizing others.

5. **Enforce Boundaries Consistently:** Enforce your boundaries consistently and assertively when they are violated or disregarded by others. Be firm in asserting your boundaries and advocating for your well-being and autonomy.

6. **Respect Others' Boundaries:** Respect the boundaries of others in your relationships, honoring their needs, preferences, and limits. Avoid crossing or disregarding others' boundaries and seek mutual understanding and respect.

7. **Set Consequences for Boundary Violations:** Set consequences for boundary violations in relationships, clearly communicating the repercussions of disregarding your boundaries. Follow through on consequences when necessary to reinforce your boundaries.

8. **Reevaluate Boundaries Regularly:** Reevaluate your boundaries regularly to ensure that they are aligned with your evolving needs and values. Adjust boundaries as needed to maintain healthy and respectful relationships.

Guidance: Set healthy boundaries in relationships by understanding their importance, reflecting on boundary violations, clarifying personal boundaries, communicating boundaries assertively, enforcing boundaries consistently, respecting others' boundaries, setting consequences for violations, and reevaluating boundaries regularly.

Cultivating Positive Relationships

Description: This worksheet focuses on cultivating positive relationships that contribute to your well-being and support your recovery journey.

Time: Set aside 20-30 minutes for this activity.

Activities:

1. **Reflect on Relationship Quality:** Reflect on the quality of your current relationships, considering how they contribute to your well-being and recovery. Identify relationships that are positive, supportive, and nurturing.
2. **Assess Relationship Dynamics:** Assess the dynamics and patterns of your relationships, considering communication styles, levels of trust, and mutual support. Identify areas where improvements can be made to enhance relationship quality.
3. **Nurture Supportive Connections:** Nurture supportive connections and relationships that align with your values and support your recovery goals. Invest time and effort in relationships that contribute positively to your well-being.
4. **Express Appreciation:** Express appreciation and gratitude to those who support you in your recovery journey. Acknowledge their contributions and the positive impact they have on your life.

5. **Set Relationship Goals:** Set specific and achievable goals for improving the quality of your relationships. Focus on areas such as communication, trust-building, and mutual support.
6. **Practice Active Listening:** Practice active listening skills in your interactions with others, focusing on understanding their perspectives, feelings, and needs. Show genuine interest and empathy in their experiences.
7. **Resolve Conflict Constructively:** Learn to resolve conflicts and disagreements constructively in your relationships, focusing on finding mutually beneficial solutions and maintaining respect and understanding.
8. **Celebrate Relationship Milestones:** Celebrate milestones and achievements in your relationships, recognizing the progress made and the growth experienced together. Use these moments to strengthen your bond and deepen your connection.

Guidance: Cultivate positive relationships by reflecting on relationship quality, assessing relationship dynamics, nurturing supportive connections, expressing appreciation, setting relationship goals, practicing active listening, resolving conflict constructively, and celebrating relationship milestones.

Strengthening Family Relationships

Description: This worksheet assists individuals in strengthening family relationships, fostering understanding, communication, and support within the family unit.

Time: Allocate 20-30 minutes for this activity.

Activities:

1. **Reflect on Family Dynamics:** Reflect on the dynamics and patterns of your family relationships, considering communication styles, roles, and interactions. Identify strengths and challenges in your family dynamics.
2. **Assess Relationship Quality:** Assess the quality of your family relationships, considering the level of trust, support, and understanding present. Identify areas where improvements can be made to strengthen family connections.
3. **Communicate Openly:** Communicate openly and honestly with family members, sharing your thoughts, feelings, and needs authentically. Foster a culture of open communication and mutual respect within the family.
4. **Express Appreciation:** Express appreciation and gratitude to your family members for their support and contributions to your life. Acknowledge their efforts and the positive impact they have on your well-being.

5. **Set Boundaries:** Set clear and appropriate boundaries with family members to protect your well-being and maintain healthy relationships. Communicate your boundaries assertively and enforce them consistently.
6. **Resolve Conflict Constructively:** Learn to resolve conflicts and disagreements constructively within the family, focusing on finding mutually acceptable solutions and maintaining respect and understanding.
7. **Share Goals and Aspirations:** Share your goals, aspirations, and recovery journey with your family members, involving them in your progress and seeking their support. Foster a sense of unity and collaboration in working towards common goals.
8. **Spend Quality Time Together:** Spend quality time together as a family, engaging in activities and conversations that promote connection and bonding. Create opportunities for meaningful interactions and shared experiences.

Guidance: Strengthen family relationships by reflecting on family dynamics, assessing relationship quality, communicating openly, expressing appreciation, setting boundaries, resolving conflict constructively, sharing goals and aspirations, and spending quality time together.

Establishing Healthy Friendships

Description: This worksheet helps individuals establish healthy friendships that support their recovery journey and contribute to their overall well-being.

Time: Set aside 20-30 minutes for this activity.

Activities:

1. **Reflect on Friendship Patterns:** Reflect on past friendship patterns and dynamics, considering how they influenced your well-being and recovery journey. Identify qualities of healthy friendships to seek out.
2. **Assess Friendship Quality:** Assess the quality of your current friendships, considering levels of trust, support, and mutual respect. Identify friendships that are positive, supportive, and nurturing.
3. **Clarify Friendship Values:** Clarify your values and priorities in friendships, considering what qualities you seek in healthy connections. Align your friendship values with your recovery goals and personal aspirations.
4. **Set Boundaries:** Set clear and appropriate boundaries in your friendships to protect your well-being and maintain healthy connections. Communicate your boundaries assertively and enforce them consistently.
5. **Seek Supportive Connections:** Seek out supportive connections and friendships that align with your

values and support your recovery journey. Surround yourself with individuals who encourage your growth and well-being.

6. **Communicate Openly:** Communicate openly and honestly with your friends, sharing your thoughts, feelings, and needs authentically. Foster a culture of open communication and mutual respect in your friendships.

7. **Share Activities and Hobbies:** Share activities and hobbies with your friends that promote connection, enjoyment, and personal growth. Engage in shared interests and experiences that strengthen your bond and deepen your connection.

8. **Be a Supportive Friend:** Be a supportive and reliable friend to others, offering encouragement, empathy, and assistance when needed. Show genuine interest and concern for your friends' well-being and success.

Guidance: Establish healthy friendships by reflecting on friendship patterns, assessing friendship quality, clarifying friendship values, setting boundaries, seeking supportive connections, communicating openly, sharing activities and hobbies, and being a supportive friend.

Fostering Supportive Relationships

Description: This worksheet focuses on fostering supportive relationships that contribute to your well-being and recovery journey.

Time: Allocate 20-30 minutes for this activity.

Activities:

1. **Reflect on Supportive Relationships:** Reflect on past experiences of supportive relationships, considering how they impacted your well-being and recovery. Identify qualities and behaviors of supportive individuals.
2. **Assess Relationship Support:** Assess the level of support available to you from current relationships, considering emotional support, practical assistance, and encouragement. Identify relationships that offer meaningful support.
3. **Express Gratitude:** Express gratitude and appreciation to supportive individuals in your life for their contributions to your well-being and recovery journey. Acknowledge their efforts and the positive impact they have had on your life.
4. **Communicate Needs:** Communicate your needs and preferences to supportive individuals in your network, being open and honest about your recovery journey and seeking their support. Express gratitude for their understanding and assistance.
5. **Offer Support in Return:** Offer support and encouragement to others in your network,

reciprocating the kindness and assistance you have received. Be a reliable and compassionate source of support for those in need.

6. **Stay Connected:** Stay connected with supportive individuals in your network, maintaining regular contact and nurturing your relationships. Cultivate meaningful connections based on mutual understanding and respect.

7. **Celebrate Achievements Together:** Celebrate achievements and milestones together with your supportive network, recognizing progress and growth. Share successes and joys with those who have supported you along the way.

Guidance: Foster supportive relationships by reflecting on supportive experiences, assessing relationship support, expressing gratitude, communicating needs, offering support in return, staying connected, and celebrating achievements together.

Seeking Healthy Social Connections

Description: This worksheet assists individuals in seeking healthy social connections and fostering a sense of belonging and community support in their recovery journey.

Time: Set aside 20-30 minutes for this activity.

Activities:

1. **Understand Social Connections:** Understand the importance of social connections in recovery, including emotional support, encouragement, and a sense of belonging. Recognize that healthy social connections contribute to well-being and resilience.
2. **Reflect on Social Needs:** Reflect on your social needs and preferences, considering the types of connections and relationships that are meaningful to you. Identify activities and settings where you feel comfortable and accepted.
3. **Assess Social Opportunities:** Assess the social opportunities available to you in your community, considering support groups, clubs, classes, and events. Identify opportunities for meeting new people and expanding your social network.
4. **Seek Out Supportive Communities:** Seek out supportive communities and groups that align with your interests and values. Join support groups, recovery meetings, or community organizations where you can connect with others who share similar experiences and goals.
5. **Participate Actively:** Participate actively in social activities and events, engaging with others and contributing positively to the community. Be open to meeting new people and building connections based on shared interests and experiences.
6. **Initiate Conversations:** Initiate conversations and interactions with others, showing genuine interest and curiosity in their experiences and perspectives.

Be approachable and friendly, and be willing to share your own story and journey.

7. **Practice Inclusivity:** Practice inclusivity and acceptance in your social interactions, welcoming diversity and respecting differences among individuals. Create a welcoming and supportive environment for everyone to feel included and valued.

8. **Nurture Connections:** Nurture connections and relationships over time, investing time and effort in building and maintaining meaningful connections. Stay connected with supportive individuals and communities that contribute positively to your recovery journey.

Guidance: Seek healthy social connections by understanding their importance, reflecting on social needs, assessing social opportunities, seeking out supportive communities, participating actively, initiating conversations, practicing inclusivity, and nurturing connections.

Balancing Social and Solitary Activities

Description: This worksheet helps individuals balance social and solitary activities in their lives, fostering a sense of connection and fulfillment while maintaining autonomy and self-care.

Time: Allocate 20-30 minutes for this activity.

Activities:

1. **Understand Activity Balance:** Understand the importance of balancing social and solitary activities in maintaining well-being and fulfillment. Recognize that both social interactions and alone time contribute to overall happiness and satisfaction.

2. **Reflect on Activity Preferences:** Reflect on your activity preferences and needs, considering the types of activities that energize and fulfill you. Identify social activities that you enjoy as well as solitary activities that recharge and rejuvenate you.

3. **Assess Current Activity Balance:** Assess the balance of social and solitary activities in your life, considering how much time and energy you devote to each. Identify areas where adjustments may be needed to achieve a healthier balance.

4. **Identify Benefits of Social Activities:** Identify the benefits of engaging in social activities, including connection, support, and a sense of belonging. Recognize the positive impact of social interactions on your mood and well-being.

5. **Recognize Benefits of Solitary Activities:** Recognize the benefits of engaging in solitary activities, including self-reflection, relaxation, and creativity. Acknowledge the importance of alone time for self-care and personal growth.

6. **Set Activity Goals:** Set specific and achievable goals for balancing social and solitary activities in your life. Consider scheduling regular social outings as well as designated time for solitude and self-care.

7. **Plan Social Interactions:** Plan social interactions and activities that align with your interests and preferences. Reach out to friends, family, or community groups to schedule gatherings or outings that promote connection and enjoyment.
8. **Schedule Solitary Time:** Schedule regular time for solitary activities and self-care practices that nurture your well-being. Prioritize activities such as reading, meditation, or hobbies that replenish your energy and promote relaxation.

Guidance: Balance social and solitary activities by understanding their importance, reflecting on activity preferences, assessing current activity balance, identifying benefits of social and solitary activities, setting activity goals, planning social interactions, and scheduling solitary time.

Setting Relationship Boundaries

Description: This worksheet assists individuals in setting relationship boundaries that protect their well-being and autonomy while fostering healthy connections with others.

Time: Set aside 20-30 minutes for this activity.

Activities:

1. **Understand Relationship Boundaries:** Understand the concept of relationship boundaries and their importance in maintaining healthy connections. Recognize that boundaries define the limits and

123

expectations of acceptable behavior in relationships.

2. **Reflect on Past Boundary Experiences:** Reflect on past experiences with relationship boundaries, considering times when boundaries were respected or violated. Identify the impact of boundary violations on your well-being and relationships.

3. **Clarify Personal Boundaries:** Clarify your personal boundaries and limits in various relationships, considering physical, emotional, and social boundaries. Identify behaviors or actions that are acceptable or unacceptable to you.

4. **Communicate Boundaries Assertively:** Communicate your boundaries assertively and respectfully to others, expressing your needs, preferences, and limits clearly and directly. Use "I" statements to convey your boundaries without blaming or criticizing others.

5. **Enforce Boundaries Consistently:** Enforce your boundaries consistently and assertively when they are violated or disregarded by others. Be firm in asserting your boundaries and advocating for your well-being and autonomy.

6. **Respect Others' Boundaries:** Respect the boundaries of others in your relationships, honoring their needs, preferences, and limits. Avoid crossing or disregarding others' boundaries and seek mutual understanding and respect.

7. **Set Consequences for Boundary Violations:** Set consequences for boundary violations in

relationships, clearly communicating the repercussions of disregarding your boundaries. Follow through on consequences when necessary to reinforce your boundaries.

8. **Reevaluate Boundaries Regularly:** Reevaluate your boundaries regularly to ensure that they are aligned with your evolving needs and values. Adjust boundaries as needed to maintain healthy and respectful relationships.

Guidance: Set relationship boundaries by understanding their importance, reflecting on boundary experiences, clarifying personal boundaries, communicating boundaries assertively, enforcing boundaries consistently, respecting others' boundaries, setting consequences for violations, and reevaluating boundaries regularly.

Strengthening Emotional Connections

Description: This worksheet focuses on strengthening emotional connections in relationships, fostering intimacy, empathy, and mutual understanding with others.

Time: Allocate 20-30 minutes for this activity.

Activities:

1. **Understand Emotional Connections:** Understand the importance of emotional connections in relationships, including intimacy, empathy, and mutual understanding. Recognize that emotional

connections contribute to the depth and quality of relationships.

2. **Reflect on Emotional Needs:** Reflect on your emotional needs and preferences in relationships, considering the types of connections and interactions that fulfill and nourish you. Identify activities and behaviors that promote emotional closeness.

3. **Assess Emotional Connections:** Assess the level of emotional connection present in your current relationships, considering the depth of intimacy, empathy, and understanding. Identify areas where improvements can be made to strengthen emotional bonds.

4. **Communicate Emotions Openly:** Communicate your emotions openly and honestly with others, sharing your thoughts, feelings, and vulnerabilities authentically. Foster a culture of emotional honesty and vulnerability in your relationships.

5. **Express Empathy and Understanding:** Express empathy and understanding towards others' experiences and emotions, validating their feelings and perspectives. Demonstrate empathy as a way of building connection and trust with others.

6. **Practice Active Listening:** Practice active listening skills in your interactions with others, focusing on understanding their perspectives, feelings, and needs. Show genuine interest and empathy in their experiences.

7. **Share Vulnerabilities:** Share your vulnerabilities and insecurities with trusted individuals in your relationships, allowing yourself to be open and authentic. Create a safe and supportive space for emotional expression and connection.

8. **Celebrate Emotional Milestones:** Celebrate emotional milestones and breakthroughs in your relationships, recognizing moments of growth and deepening connection. Share joys and challenges together as a way of strengthening emotional bonds.

Guidance: Strengthen emotional connections by understanding their importance, reflecting on emotional needs, assessing emotional connections, communicating emotions openly, expressing empathy and understanding, practicing active listening, sharing vulnerabilities, and celebrating emotional milestones.

Fostering Intimacy in Relationships

Description: This worksheet assists individuals in fostering intimacy in relationships, cultivating closeness, trust, and vulnerability with others.

Time: Set aside 20-30 minutes for this activity.

Activities:

1. **Understand Intimacy:** Understand the concept of intimacy and its importance in relationships, including emotional closeness, trust, and

vulnerability. Recognize that intimacy deepens connection and strengthens relationships.

2. **Reflect on Intimacy Needs:** Reflect on your intimacy needs and preferences in relationships, considering the types of connections and interactions that foster closeness and vulnerability. Identify activities and behaviors that promote intimacy.

3. **Assess Intimacy Levels:** Assess the level of intimacy present in your current relationships, considering the depth of emotional connection, trust, and vulnerability. Identify areas where improvements can be made to enhance intimacy.

4. **Communicate Openly:** Communicate openly and honestly with others about your desire for intimacy and closeness in relationships. Express your thoughts, feelings, and vulnerabilities authentically, fostering emotional honesty and vulnerability.

5. **Express Affection:** Express affection and appreciation towards others in your relationships, showing care, compassion, and love. Demonstrate your feelings through words, gestures, and actions that promote closeness and connection.

6. **Share Personal Stories:** Share personal stories and experiences with trusted individuals in your relationships, allowing yourself to be open and vulnerable. Create a safe and supportive space for sharing and listening to each other's stories.

7. **Practice Trust-Building:** Practice trust-building behaviors and actions in your relationships,

demonstrating reliability, honesty, and integrity. Build trust over time through consistent and respectful interactions.

8. **Celebrate Relationship Milestones:** Celebrate relationship milestones and moments of intimacy together, recognizing the progress made and the growth experienced. Use these moments to deepen connection and strengthen bonds.

Guidance: Foster intimacy in relationships by understanding its importance, reflecting on intimacy needs, assessing intimacy levels, communicating openly, expressing affection, sharing personal stories, practicing trust-building, and celebrating relationship milestones.

Enhancing Interpersonal Skills

Description: This worksheet focuses on enhancing interpersonal skills, including communication, empathy, and conflict resolution, to improve relationships with others.

Time: Allocate 20-30 minutes for this activity.

Activities:

1. **Understand Interpersonal Skills:** Understand the importance of interpersonal skills in building and maintaining relationships, including communication, empathy, and conflict resolution. Recognize that interpersonal skills contribute to effective and meaningful interactions.

2. **Reflect on Interpersonal Strengths:** Reflect on your strengths and areas for improvement in interpersonal skills, considering past experiences and interactions with others. Identify skills that you excel in and areas where you can grow.

3. **Assess Communication Styles:** Assess your communication style and its impact on your relationships, considering factors such as clarity, assertiveness, and active listening. Identify communication patterns that contribute to positive or negative interactions.

4. **Practice Active Listening:** Practice active listening skills in your interactions with others, focusing on understanding their perspectives, feelings, and needs. Listen attentively without interrupting or judging, and paraphrase to ensure understanding.

5. **Express Thoughts and Feelings:** Express your thoughts and feelings assertively and respectfully during interactions, using "I" statements to convey your perspective. Avoid blaming or criticizing others and focus on expressing your own needs and concerns.

6. **Demonstrate Empathy:** Demonstrate empathy and understanding towards others' experiences and emotions, validating their feelings and perspectives. Show compassion and support in your interactions to foster connection and trust.

7. **Resolve Conflict Constructively:** Learn to resolve conflicts and disagreements constructively in your relationships, focusing on finding mutually

beneficial solutions and maintaining respect and understanding.

8. **Seek Feedback and Guidance:** Seek feedback and guidance from trusted individuals in improving your interpersonal skills, asking for specific examples and suggestions for growth. Use feedback as a tool for self-awareness and improvement.

Guidance: Enhance interpersonal skills by understanding their importance, reflecting on strengths and areas for improvement, assessing communication styles, practicing active listening, expressing thoughts and feelings assertively, demonstrating empathy, resolving conflict constructively, and seeking feedback and guidance.

Building Healthy Communication Patterns

Description: This worksheet assists individuals in building healthy communication patterns in relationships, fostering understanding, respect, and connection with others.

Time: Set aside 20-30 minutes for this activity.

Activities:

1. **Understand Communication Patterns:** Understand the importance of communication patterns in relationships, including clarity, respect, and active listening. Recognize that healthy communication fosters understanding and connection with others.

2. **Reflect on Communication Styles:** Reflect on your communication style and its impact on your

relationships, considering factors such as clarity, assertiveness, and empathy. Identify communication patterns that contribute to positive or negative interactions.

3. **Assess Communication Dynamics:** Assess the communication dynamics present in your relationships, considering the level of openness, honesty, and mutual respect. Identify areas where improvements can be made to enhance communication.

4. **Practice Active Listening:** Practice active listening skills in your interactions with others, focusing on understanding their perspectives, feelings, and needs. Listen attentively without interrupting or judging, and paraphrase to ensure understanding.

5. **Express Thoughts and Feelings:** Express your thoughts and feelings assertively and respectfully during interactions, using "I" statements to convey your perspective. Avoid blaming or criticizing others and focus on expressing your own needs and concerns.

6. **Show Empathy and Understanding:** Show empathy and understanding towards others' experiences and emotions, validating their feelings and perspectives. Demonstrate compassion and support to foster connection and trust.

7. **Set Clear Expectations:** Set clear expectations for communication in your relationships, establishing guidelines for respectful and effective interaction.

Encourage openness and honesty in expressing thoughts and feelings.

8. **Resolve Misunderstandings Promptly:** Learn to resolve misunderstandings and conflicts promptly in your relationships, addressing issues directly and constructively. Focus on finding solutions and maintaining respect and understanding.

Guidance: Build healthy communication patterns by understanding their importance, reflecting on communication styles, assessing communication dynamics, practicing active listening, expressing thoughts and feelings assertively, showing empathy and understanding, setting clear expectations, and resolving misunderstandings promptly.

Section 3: Coping Strategies

Section 3 focuses on providing individuals with practical tools and techniques to manage the challenges and stressors they may encounter during their recovery journey from substance abuse. This section is designed to equip individuals with effective coping skills that can help them navigate cravings, triggers, and difficult emotions without resorting to substance use.

Stress Management Techniques

Description: This worksheet introduces stress management techniques, including mindfulness, deep breathing, and progressive muscle relaxation, to promote relaxation and reduce stress levels.

Time: Allocate 15-20 minutes for this activity.

Activities:

1. **Mindfulness Meditation:** Practice mindfulness meditation by focusing on your breath and observing thoughts without judgment. Allow yourself to be fully present in the moment.
2. **Deep Breathing Exercise:** Practice deep breathing exercises to calm the nervous system and reduce stress. Inhale deeply through your nose, hold for a few seconds, and exhale slowly through your mouth.
3. **Progressive Muscle Relaxation:** Tense and relax each muscle group in your body, starting from your toes and working your way up to your head. Notice the difference between tension and relaxation.
4. **Body Scan Meditation:** Perform a body scan meditation by systematically directing your attention to different parts of your body, noticing sensations without trying to change them.
5. **Visualization:** Use visualization techniques to imagine yourself in a peaceful and serene environment. Picture yourself surrounded by

calming elements, such as nature or soothing colors.

6. **Guided Imagery:** Listen to a guided imagery recording or create your own visualization script to guide you through a relaxation journey.

7. **Breath Counting:** Count your breaths as you inhale and exhale, focusing on the rhythm and pace of your breathing. Gradually lengthen your exhale to promote relaxation.

Guidance: Practice stress management techniques regularly to promote relaxation and reduce stress levels. Experiment with different techniques to find what works best for you.

Therapist Tips:

- Encourage clients to integrate stress management techniques into their daily routines, especially during times of increased stress.
- Remind clients that consistency is key when practicing stress management techniques, and encourage them to be patient with themselves as they develop these skills.
- Emphasize the importance of self-care and encourage clients to prioritize their mental and emotional well-being.

Assertiveness Training

Description: This worksheet provides exercises to practice assertive communication skills in various scenarios, empowering individuals to express their needs and boundaries effectively.

Time: Set aside 20-30 minutes for this activity.

Activities:

1. **Identify Assertive Behaviors:** Identify assertive behaviors, such as expressing opinions respectfully, setting boundaries, and standing up for yourself without aggression or passivity.
2. **Role-Playing Scenarios:** Role-play various scenarios where assertive communication is required, such as expressing disagreement with a friend or colleague, declining a request, or asking for help.
3. **Assertiveness Scripts:** Develop assertiveness scripts for challenging situations, outlining what you will say and how you will communicate your needs assertively.
4. **Positive Affirmations:** Practice positive affirmations to boost confidence and self-esteem, reinforcing your right to assert yourself and express your needs.
5. **Body Language Awareness:** Pay attention to your body language during interactions, ensuring it reflects assertiveness and confidence. Maintain eye

contact, use open and relaxed gestures, and stand or sit upright.

6. **Setting Boundaries:** Practice setting clear and respectful boundaries in your relationships and interactions with others. Communicate your boundaries assertively and enforce them consistently.

7. **Self-Reflection:** Reflect on past experiences where you were assertive and the positive outcomes that resulted from expressing yourself confidently and respectfully.

Guidance: Practice assertiveness training exercises regularly to enhance communication skills and build confidence in expressing your needs and boundaries.

Therapist Tips:

- Encourage clients to start with small, low-risk situations when practicing assertiveness and gradually work up to more challenging scenarios.
- Remind clients that assertiveness is a skill that can be learned and developed over time with practice and persistence.
- Validate clients' experiences and reassure them that it's normal to feel uncomfortable or anxious when first practicing assertive communication. Encourage them to acknowledge their feelings and continue practicing.

Problem-Solving Skills

Description: This worksheet provides a step-by-step guide to identifying and solving problems without resorting to substance use, empowering individuals to effectively manage challenges.

Time: Allocate 20-30 minutes for this activity.

Activities:

1. **Identify the Problem:** Clearly define the problem you are facing, being specific about what needs to be addressed.
2. **Brainstorm Solutions:** Generate a list of possible solutions to the problem, considering a range of options without judgment.
3. **Evaluate Solutions:** Evaluate each solution based on its feasibility, potential outcomes, and alignment with your values and goals.
4. **Select a Solution:** Choose the most promising solution from your list, considering its likelihood of success and potential impact on the situation.
5. **Develop an Action Plan:** Create a step-by-step action plan for implementing the chosen solution, breaking down the process into manageable tasks.
6. **Implement the Plan:** Put your action plan into action, taking concrete steps to address the problem and work towards a resolution.

7. **Monitor Progress:** Monitor your progress as you work through the action plan, adjusting strategies as needed and staying flexible in your approach.

8. **Reflect on Outcomes:** Reflect on the outcomes of your problem-solving efforts, considering what worked well and what could be improved for future challenges.

Guidance: Use problem-solving skills to effectively address challenges and overcome obstacles without resorting to substance use. Focus on breaking down problems, brainstorming solutions, evaluating options, and taking action.

Therapist Tips:

- Encourage clients to approach problem-solving with a proactive and solution-focused mindset, focusing on what they can control rather than dwelling on obstacles.
- Remind clients that setbacks and challenges are a normal part of the problem-solving process and encourage them to view them as opportunities for growth and learning.
- Offer guidance and support as clients work through the problem-solving process, providing encouragement and validation of their efforts.

Developing Healthy Habits

Description: This worksheet provides exercises for establishing routines and incorporating healthy activities into daily life, promoting overall well-being and resilience.

Time: Set aside 15-20 minutes for this activity.

Activities:

1. **Identify Areas for Improvement:** Identify areas of your life where you would like to establish healthier habits, such as sleep, nutrition, exercise, and self-care.

2. **Set SMART Goals:** Set specific, measurable, achievable, relevant, and time-bound (SMART) goals for developing healthy habits in each area identified.

3. **Create a Daily Routine:** Create a daily routine that includes time for healthy activities, such as exercise, meal preparation, relaxation, and self-care.

4. **Prioritize Self-Care:** Prioritize self-care activities that nurture your physical, emotional, and mental well-being, such as meditation, journaling, or spending time outdoors.

5. **Monitor Progress:** Keep track of your progress towards developing healthy habits, using a journal or habit-tracking app to monitor your actions and identify areas for improvement.

6. **Celebrate Achievements:** Celebrate your achievements and milestones along the way, acknowledging the progress you've made towards establishing healthier habits.

7. **Stay Flexible:** Remain flexible and adaptable in your approach to developing healthy habits, recognizing that setbacks and challenges are a normal part of the process.

8. **Seek Support:** Seek support from friends, family, or professionals as needed, and surround yourself with individuals who encourage and support your efforts to live a healthier lifestyle.

Guidance: Use the exercises in this worksheet to develop healthy habits that support your overall well-being and resilience. Focus on setting goals, creating routines, prioritizing self-care, monitoring progress, celebrating achievements, staying flexible, and seeking support.

Therapist Tips:

- Encourage clients to start small and gradually build upon their healthy habits over time, focusing on sustainable changes that fit their lifestyle.
- Remind clients that developing healthy habits is a process that requires patience, consistency, and self-compassion. Encourage them to be gentle with themselves and to celebrate their progress along the way.
- Offer guidance and support as clients work towards developing healthy habits, providing

encouragement, accountability, and practical strategies for overcoming obstacles.

Relaxation Techniques

Description: This worksheet introduces various relaxation techniques to reduce stress and promote a sense of calmness and well-being.

Time: Allocate 20-30 minutes for this activity.

Activities:

1. **Progressive Muscle Relaxation:** Practice tensing and relaxing different muscle groups in your body, starting from your toes and working your way up to your head. Focus on releasing tension and promoting relaxation.
2. **Guided Imagery:** Listen to a guided imagery recording or create your own visualization script to guide you through a relaxation journey. Imagine yourself in a peaceful and serene environment.
3. **Breath Counting:** Count your breaths as you inhale and exhale, focusing on the rhythm and pace of your breathing. Gradually lengthen your exhale to promote relaxation and calmness.
4. **Body Scan Meditation:** Perform a body scan meditation by systematically directing your attention to different parts of your body, noticing sensations without trying to change them. Allow yourself to relax and let go of tension.

5. **Nature Sounds:** Listen to recordings of nature sounds, such as ocean waves, birdsong, or rainfall, to create a calming and tranquil atmosphere.

6. **Aromatherapy:** Use essential oils or scented candles with relaxing fragrances, such as lavender or chamomile, to create a soothing environment and promote relaxation.

7. **Mindful Walking:** Practice mindful walking by paying attention to each step you take, noticing sensations in your feet and legs as they make contact with the ground. Allow yourself to be fully present in the act of walking.

8. **Progressive Relaxation Script:** Create a progressive relaxation script that guides you through the process of relaxing each muscle group in your body. Record yourself reading the script or ask a friend to read it aloud to you.

Guidance: Use relaxation techniques regularly to reduce stress, promote relaxation, and enhance overall well-being. Experiment with different techniques to find what works best for you.

Therapist Tips:

- Encourage clients to incorporate relaxation techniques into their daily routines, especially during times of heightened stress or tension.
- Remind clients that relaxation is a skill that can be developed with practice, and encourage them to be

patient with themselves as they explore different techniques.

- Offer guidance and support as clients experiment with relaxation techniques, providing encouragement and validation of their efforts.

Coping with Triggers

Description: This worksheet helps individuals identify triggers for substance use and develop coping strategies to manage cravings and avoid relapse.

Time: Set aside 20-30 minutes for this activity.

Activities:

1. **Identify Triggers:** Identify common triggers for substance use, such as stress, negative emotions, social situations, or environmental cues.
2. **Develop Coping Strategies:** Brainstorm healthy coping strategies to manage cravings and avoid relapse when faced with triggers. Focus on strategies that address the underlying reasons for substance use.
3. **Create a Coping Plan:** Develop a coping plan that outlines specific steps to take when encountering triggers. Include coping strategies, support resources, and emergency contacts.
4. **Practice Self-Care:** Prioritize self-care activities that nurture your physical, emotional, and mental well-being, reducing vulnerability to triggers and cravings.

5. **Seek Support:** Reach out to friends, family, or support groups for encouragement and guidance when facing triggers. Share your coping plan with trusted individuals who can offer support and accountability.

6. **Mindfulness Practice:** Practice mindfulness techniques to increase awareness of cravings and trigger cues without reacting impulsively. Observe thoughts and sensations nonjudgmentally.

7. **Distraction Strategies:** Engage in distracting activities to shift your focus away from cravings and triggers. Choose activities that are enjoyable, absorbing, and incompatible with substance use.

8. **Healthy Alternatives:** Explore healthy alternatives to substance use that provide similar benefits or rewards. Find activities that fulfill emotional needs and promote well-being without negative consequences.

Guidance: Use this worksheet to develop coping strategies for managing triggers and cravings, reducing the risk of relapse, and maintaining sobriety.

Therapist Tips:

- Encourage clients to practice coping strategies regularly, even during times of stability, to strengthen their ability to manage triggers effectively.

- Remind clients that relapse is a common part of the recovery process and encourage them to view setbacks as opportunities for learning and growth.
- Offer support and guidance as clients develop their coping plans, providing validation and encouragement of their efforts to maintain sobriety.

Emotional Regulation Technique

Description: This worksheet provides techniques to regulate emotions and cope with intense feelings in healthy ways.

Time: Allocate 15-20 minutes for this activity.

Activities:

1. **Identify Emotions:** Identify and label your emotions accurately, recognizing the physical sensations and thoughts associated with each emotion.
2. **Deep Breathing:** Practice deep breathing exercises to calm the nervous system and reduce emotional arousal. Inhale deeply through your nose, hold for a few seconds, and exhale slowly through your mouth.
3. **Mindfulness Meditation:** Practice mindfulness meditation to cultivate present moment awareness and reduce emotional reactivity. Focus on your breath or bodily sensations and observe thoughts without judgment.

4. **Positive Self-Talk:** Challenge negative thoughts and replace them with positive affirmations. Offer yourself words of encouragement and support.
5. **Grounding Techniques:** Use grounding techniques, such as the 5-4-3-2-1 method or progressive muscle relaxation, to anchor yourself in the present moment and reduce emotional distress.
6. **Journaling:** Write about your emotions in a journal, expressing your thoughts and feelings freely. Use writing as a tool for self-reflection and emotional processing.
7. **Creative Expression:** Engage in creative outlets, such as art, music, or dance, as a means of expressing and processing emotions.
8. **Seek Support:** Reach out to friends, family, or mental health professionals for support and validation when experiencing intense emotions.

Guidance: Use emotional regulation techniques to cope with intense feelings and promote emotional well-being. Focus on identifying emotions, practicing deep breathing and mindfulness, challenging negative thoughts, using grounding techniques, journaling, engaging in creative expression, and seeking support.

Therapist Tips:

- Encourage clients to practice emotional regulation techniques regularly to enhance emotional resilience and coping skills.

- Remind clients that emotions are a normal and natural part of the human experience, and it's okay to feel a wide range of emotions.
- Offer validation and support as clients explore and express their emotions, providing a safe and nonjudgmental space for emotional processing.

Cognitive Restructuring

Description: This worksheet introduces cognitive restructuring techniques to challenge and modify negative thought patterns.

Time: Set aside 20-30 minutes for this activity.

Activities:

1. **Identify Negative Thoughts:** Identify and write down negative thoughts or beliefs that contribute to distressing emotions.
2. **Evaluate Evidence:** Evaluate the evidence for and against the negative thoughts, considering objective facts and alternative interpretations.
3. **Challenge Irrational Beliefs:** Challenge irrational beliefs and cognitive distortions, such as black-and-white thinking, catastrophizing, or overgeneralization.
4. **Generate Alternative Thoughts:** Generate alternative, more balanced thoughts that are realistic and evidence-based. Consider different perspectives and reinterpretations of the situation.

5. **Practice Positive Self-Talk:** Practice positive self-talk and affirmations to counteract negative thoughts and promote self-esteem and self-confidence.
6. **Reframe Negative Situations:** Reframe negative situations as opportunities for growth and learning. Focus on what you can control and how you can adapt and overcome challenges.
7. **Visualize Success:** Visualize yourself overcoming obstacles and achieving your goals. Use imagery and visualization techniques to reinforce positive beliefs and outcomes.
8. **Seek Support:** Seek support from friends, family, or mental health professionals for additional perspective and validation when challenging negative thoughts.

Guidance: Use cognitive restructuring techniques to challenge and modify negative thought patterns, promoting a more balanced and adaptive mindset. Focus on identifying negative thoughts, evaluating evidence, challenging irrational beliefs, generating alternative thoughts, practicing positive self-talk, reframing negative situations, visualizing success, and seeking support.

Therapist Tips:

- Encourage clients to approach cognitive restructuring with curiosity and openness, exploring different perspectives and interpretations of situations.

- Remind clients that changing negative thought patterns takes time and practice, and encourage them to be patient and compassionate with themselves throughout the process.
- Offer guidance and support as clients challenge negative thoughts, providing validation and encouragement of their efforts to cultivate a more positive and adaptive mindset.

Distress Tolerance Techniques

Description: This worksheet introduces distress tolerance techniques to help individuals cope with overwhelming emotions and situations without resorting to harmful behaviors.

Time: Allocate 20-30 minutes for this activity.

Activities:

1. **Self-Soothing Strategies:** Practice self-soothing techniques, such as taking a warm bath, listening to calming music, or cuddling with a pet, to comfort yourself and reduce emotional distress.
2. **Distract with Activities:** Engage in activities that distract your attention from distressing thoughts and emotions, such as exercising, cooking, or doing puzzles.
3. **Opposite Action:** Act opposite to your emotions by engaging in behaviors that are the opposite of what you feel like doing. For example, if you feel like

isolating yourself, reach out to a friend or loved one for support.

4. **Improve the Moment:** Focus on improving the moment by finding small pleasures or positive aspects in your surroundings. Practice gratitude and mindfulness to increase appreciation for the present moment.

5. **TIPP Skills:** Use TIPP skills (Temperature, Intense Exercise, Paced Breathing, and Paired Muscle Relaxation) to quickly reduce emotional arousal and distress.

6. **Crisis Survival Strategies:** Develop a crisis survival plan that outlines specific steps to take when experiencing intense distress or urges to engage in harmful behaviors. Include coping strategies, support resources, and emergency contacts.

7. **Grounding Techniques:** Use grounding techniques, such as focusing on your senses or engaging in mindfulness exercises, to anchor yourself in the present moment and reduce emotional intensity.

8. **Seek Support:** Reach out to friends, family, or mental health professionals for support and validation when experiencing overwhelming emotions or situations.

Guidance: Use distress tolerance techniques to cope with overwhelming emotions and situations, reducing the risk of engaging in harmful behaviors. Focus on self-soothing strategies, distracting with activities, opposite action, improving the moment, TIPP skills, crisis survival strategies, grounding techniques, and seeking support.

Therapist Tips:

- Encourage clients to practice distress tolerance techniques regularly to build resilience and coping skills.
- Remind clients that distress tolerance is about getting through difficult moments without making them worse, not about solving problems or eliminating distress altogether.
- Offer guidance and support as clients explore and implement distress tolerance techniques, providing validation and encouragement of their efforts to cope effectively with overwhelming emotions and situations.

Anger Management Strategies

Description: This worksheet provides strategies to manage and cope with anger in healthy and constructive ways.

Time: Set aside 20-30 minutes for this activity.

Activities:

1. **Identify Anger Triggers:** Identify common triggers for anger, such as frustration, injustice, or feeling misunderstood.
2. **Recognize Early Warning Signs:** Learn to recognize early warning signs of anger, such as muscle tension, clenched fists, or racing thoughts.

3. **Pause and Breathe:** Practice pausing and taking deep breaths when you feel anger rising, allowing yourself a moment to calm down before reacting impulsively.

4. **Express Yourself Assertively:** Express your feelings assertively and directly, using "I" statements to communicate your needs and boundaries without aggression or hostility.

5. **Take a Time-Out:** Take a break from the situation if you feel overwhelmed by anger, giving yourself time to cool off and gain perspective before addressing the issue.

6. **Use Relaxation Techniques:** Use relaxation techniques, such as deep breathing, progressive muscle relaxation, or visualization, to calm your body and mind when feeling angry.

7. **Practice Problem-Solving:** Identify the underlying issues contributing to your anger and work towards finding constructive solutions to address them.

8. **Seek Support:** Reach out to friends, family, or mental health professionals for support and guidance when struggling to manage anger effectively.

Guidance: Use anger management strategies to cope with feelings of anger in healthy and constructive ways. Focus on identifying anger triggers, recognizing early warning signs, pausing and breathing, expressing yourself assertively, taking a time-out, using relaxation techniques, practicing problem-solving, and seeking support.

Therapist Tips:

- Encourage clients to practice anger management techniques regularly to build self-awareness and coping skills.
- Remind clients that anger is a normal and natural emotion, but it's important to express it in healthy and constructive ways.
- Offer guidance and support as clients navigate their anger triggers and develop strategies for managing anger effectively, providing validation and encouragement of their efforts to cope with difficult emotions.

Substance Refusal Skills

Description: This worksheet provides strategies to resist peer pressure and refuse offers of substances in social situations.

Time: Allocate 20-30 minutes for this activity.

Activities:

1. **Practice Saying No:** Practice saying no to offers of substances in various social situations, using assertive and confident body language and tone of voice.
2. **Use Assertive Communication:** Use assertive communication skills to express your refusal clearly and respectfully, without making excuses or apologizing.

3. **Provide Alternatives:** Provide alternatives to substance use in social situations, such as suggesting non-alcoholic beverages or engaging in alternative activities.
4. **Set Boundaries:** Set and communicate clear boundaries with friends and peers regarding substance use, making it known that you do not want to participate in activities involving substances.
5. **Use Delay Tactics:** Use delay tactics to give yourself time to consider your response and come up with an appropriate refusal strategy, such as saying you need to check your schedule or consult with someone else.
6. **Enlist Support:** Enlist the support of friends or allies who respect your decision to abstain from substance use and can help you navigate challenging social situations.
7. **Plan Ahead:** Plan ahead for social events by anticipating potential triggers and practicing refusal skills in advance.
8. **Seek Support:** Reach out to friends, family, or support groups for encouragement and guidance when facing peer pressure to use substances.

Guidance: Use substance refusal skills to resist peer pressure and refuse offers of substances in social situations. Focus on practicing saying no, using assertive communication, providing alternatives, setting boundaries, using delay tactics, enlisting support, planning ahead, and seeking support.

Therapist Tips:

- Encourage clients to practice substance refusal skills regularly to build confidence and assertiveness in social situations.
- Remind clients that it's okay to say no to substance use, even if others are pressuring them to participate.
- Offer guidance and support as clients navigate social situations involving substance use, providing validation and encouragement of their efforts to maintain sobriety and resist peer pressure.

Distraction Techniques

Description: This worksheet provides distraction techniques to redirect attention away from cravings or distressing thoughts.

Time: Set aside 15-20 minutes for this activity.

Activities:

1. **Engage in Physical Activity:** Take a brisk walk, go for a run, or engage in another form of exercise to distract yourself and release tension.
2. **Listen to Music:** Listen to music that uplifts your mood or energizes you, providing a welcome distraction from cravings or negative thoughts.

3. **Watch a Movie or TV Show:** Watch a movie or TV show that captures your interest and absorbs your attention, allowing you to temporarily escape from cravings or distressing thoughts.

4. **Read a Book or Magazine:** Read a book, magazine, or article on a topic that interests you, immersing yourself in the story or information to distract from cravings or negative emotions.

5. **Engage in a Hobby:** Engage in a hobby or creative activity, such as painting, gardening, or cooking, that occupies your mind and provides a sense of enjoyment and fulfillment.

6. **Socialize with Friends or Family:** Spend time with friends or family members who provide support and distraction from cravings or distressing thoughts.

7. **Play a Game:** Play a game, whether it's a board game, card game, or video game, that requires concentration and provides an entertaining distraction.

8. **Practice Mindfulness:** Practice mindfulness techniques, such as deep breathing or body scan meditation, to anchor yourself in the present moment and reduce the power of cravings or distressing thoughts.

Guidance: Use distraction techniques to redirect attention away from cravings or distressing thoughts, providing temporary relief and promoting resilience. Focus on engaging in physical activity, listening to music, watching a movie or TV show, reading a book or magazine, engaging in a hobby, socializing with friends or family, playing a game, and practicing mindfulness.

Therapist Tips:

- Encourage clients to experiment with different distraction techniques to find what works best for them in different situations.
- Remind clients that distraction techniques are a useful tool for managing cravings or distressing thoughts in the short term, but they may need to be combined with other coping strategies for long-term success.
- Offer guidance and support as clients practice distraction techniques, providing validation and encouragement of their efforts to cope with cravings or distressing thoughts effectively.

Problem-Solving Skills

Description: This worksheet introduces problem-solving skills to help individuals identify and address challenges in their lives.

Time: Allocate 20-30 minutes for this activity.

Activities:

1. **Identify the Problem:** Clearly define the problem or challenge you are facing, being specific and objective in your description.

2. **Brainstorm Solutions:** Brainstorm potential solutions to the problem, considering a wide range of possibilities without judgment or evaluation.
3. **Evaluate Solutions:** Evaluate each potential solution based on its feasibility, effectiveness, and potential consequences. Consider the pros and cons of each option.
4. **Select a Solution:** Select the solution that seems most practical, realistic, and likely to address the problem effectively. Trust your judgment and intuition.
5. **Develop an Action Plan:** Develop a step-by-step action plan for implementing the chosen solution, outlining specific tasks, deadlines, and resources needed.
6. **Implement the Plan:** Take action to implement the plan, following through on each step and adjusting as needed based on feedback and progress.
7. **Monitor Progress:** Monitor your progress as you work towards solving the problem, assessing what is working well and what may need to be adjusted.
8. **Seek Support:** Seek support from friends, family, or professionals if you encounter obstacles or need guidance along the way.

Guidance: Use problem-solving skills to identify and address challenges effectively, promoting resilience and empowerment. Focus on identifying the problem, brainstorming solutions, evaluating solutions, selecting a solution, developing an action plan, implementing the plan, monitoring progress, and seeking support.

Therapist Tips:

- Encourage clients to approach problem-solving with creativity, flexibility, and persistence, recognizing that there may be multiple ways to address a challenge.
- Remind clients that problem-solving is a skill that can be developed with practice and experience, and encourage them to be patient and persistent in their efforts.
- Offer guidance and support as clients navigate the problem-solving process, providing validation and encouragement of their efforts to overcome challenges effectively.

Emotional Regulation Strategies

Description: This worksheet provides strategies to regulate emotions and cope with intense feelings in healthy ways.

Time: Set aside 20-30 minutes for this activity.

Activities:

1. **Identify Emotions:** Identify and label your emotions accurately, recognizing the physical sensations and thoughts associated with each emotion.
2. **Practice Deep Breathing:** Practice deep breathing exercises to calm the nervous system and reduce

emotional arousal. Inhale deeply through your nose, hold for a few seconds, and exhale slowly through your mouth.

3. **Use Grounding Techniques:** Use grounding techniques, such as focusing on your senses or engaging in mindfulness exercises, to anchor yourself in the present moment and reduce emotional intensity.

4. **Engage in Self-Compassion:** Practice self-compassion by offering yourself kindness, understanding, and acceptance during times of emotional distress.

5. **Express Emotions Creatively:** Express your emotions creatively through art, music, writing, or other forms of creative expression, allowing yourself to process and release intense feelings.

6. **Seek Social Support:** Reach out to friends, family, or support groups for validation and empathy when experiencing intense emotions, sharing your feelings and seeking comfort.

7. **Practice Mindfulness:** Practice mindfulness techniques, such as body scan meditation or mindful breathing, to cultivate present moment awareness and reduce emotional reactivity.

8. **Use Cognitive Restructuring:** Use cognitive restructuring techniques to challenge and modify negative thought patterns that contribute to emotional distress.

Guidance: Use emotional regulation strategies to cope with intense feelings and promote emotional well-being. Focus on identifying emotions, practicing deep breathing, using grounding techniques, engaging in self-compassion, expressing emotions creatively, seeking social support, practicing mindfulness, and using cognitive restructuring.

Therapist Tips:

- Encourage clients to practice emotional regulation strategies regularly to build resilience and coping skills.
- Remind clients that emotions are a natural and normal part of the human experience, and it's important to acknowledge and express them in healthy ways.
- Offer guidance and support as clients navigate intense emotions, providing validation and encouragement of their efforts to regulate emotions effectively.

Time Management Skills

Description: This worksheet introduces time management skills to help individuals prioritize tasks, set goals, and use their time effectively.

Time: Allocate 20-30 minutes for this activity.

Activities:

1. **Set SMART Goals:** Set specific, measurable, achievable, relevant, and time-bound (SMART) goals for tasks or activities you want to accomplish.
2. **Prioritize Tasks:** Prioritize tasks based on their importance and urgency, focusing on high-priority tasks that align with your goals and values.
3. **Break Tasks into Smaller Steps:** Break larger tasks into smaller, more manageable steps to make them less overwhelming and easier to tackle.
4. **Create a Schedule:** Create a daily or weekly schedule that allocates time for each task or activity, making sure to include breaks and time for self-care.
5. **Use Time Blocking:** Use time blocking techniques to allocate specific time slots for different tasks or activities, helping you stay focused and productive.
6. **Minimize Distractions:** Minimize distractions by turning off notifications, setting boundaries with others, and creating a conducive work environment.
7. **Stay Flexible:** Stay flexible and adaptable in your approach to time management, recognizing that unexpected events or changes may require adjustments to your schedule.
8. **Reflect and Adjust:** Regularly reflect on your time management practices and adjust as needed based on what is working well and what could be improved.

Guidance: Use time management skills to prioritize tasks, set goals, and use your time effectively, promoting productivity and reducing stress. Focus on setting SMART goals, prioritizing tasks, breaking tasks into smaller steps, creating a schedule, using time blocking, minimizing distractions, staying flexible, and reflecting and adjusting.

Therapist Tips:

- Encourage clients to experiment with different time management techniques to find what works best for them.
- Remind clients that effective time management is about making intentional choices about how to spend their time and aligning their actions with their goals and values.
- Offer guidance and support as clients develop and implement their time management strategies, providing validation and encouragement of their efforts to improve their productivity and well-being.

Relaxation Techniques

Description: This worksheet introduces relaxation techniques to reduce stress, promote relaxation, and improve overall well-being.

Time: Set aside 20-30 minutes for this activity.

Activities:

1. **Progressive Muscle Relaxation (PMR):** Practice PMR by systematically tensing and relaxing different muscle groups in your body, starting from your toes and working your way up to your head.
2. **Deep Breathing Exercises:** Practice deep breathing exercises to activate the body's relaxation response and reduce stress. Inhale deeply through your nose, hold for a few seconds, and exhale slowly through your mouth.
3. **Guided Imagery:** Practice guided imagery by visualizing yourself in a peaceful and calming environment, using all your senses to create a vivid mental image.
4. **Mindfulness Meditation:** Practice mindfulness meditation by focusing your attention on the present moment, observing your thoughts and sensations without judgment.
5. **Body Scan Meditation:** Practice body scan meditation by systematically scanning your body for any areas of tension or discomfort and releasing tension with each breath.
6. **Yoga or Tai Chi:** Practice yoga or tai chi, gentle and flowing movement practices that promote relaxation, flexibility, and mindfulness.
7. **Listening to Relaxing Music:** Listen to relaxing music or nature sounds that promote relaxation and reduce stress, allowing yourself to unwind and let go of tension.

8. **Engage in a Relaxing Activity:** Engage in a relaxing activity that you enjoy, such as taking a warm bath, reading a book, or spending time in nature.

Guidance: Use relaxation techniques to reduce stress, promote relaxation, and improve overall well-being. Focus on progressive muscle relaxation, deep breathing exercises, guided imagery, mindfulness meditation, body scan meditation, yoga or tai chi, listening to relaxing music, and engaging in relaxing activities.

Therapist Tips:

- Encourage clients to practice relaxation techniques regularly to build resilience and coping skills.
- Remind clients that relaxation techniques are a valuable tool for managing stress and promoting well-being, and encourage them to prioritize self-care.
- Offer guidance and support as clients explore and implement relaxation techniques, providing validation and encouragement of their efforts to reduce stress and promote relaxation.

Assertiveness Training

Description: This worksheet introduces assertiveness training exercises to help individuals communicate their needs, thoughts, and feelings effectively.

Time: Allocate 20-30 minutes for this activity.

Activities:

1. **Identify Your Rights:** Identify your rights as an individual, including the right to express your thoughts and feelings, set boundaries, and assert yourself in relationships.

2. **Practice Assertive Communication:** Practice assertive communication by expressing your needs, thoughts, and feelings directly and respectfully, using "I" statements and assertive body language.

3. **Role-Play Scenarios:** Role-play different scenarios where assertive communication may be challenging, such as setting boundaries with friends or colleagues, and practice assertive responses.

4. **Set Boundaries:** Set boundaries with others by clearly communicating your limits, saying no when necessary, and advocating for yourself assertively.

5. **Use Assertive Body Language:** Use assertive body language, such as maintaining eye contact, standing or sitting upright, and speaking clearly and confidently, to convey assertiveness.

6. **Practice Self-Validation:** Practice self-validation by acknowledging and affirming your feelings, thoughts, and experiences, even if others may not agree or understand.

7. **Handle Criticism Assertively:** Handle criticism assertively by listening non-defensively, acknowledging feedback, and expressing your perspective calmly and respectfully.

8. **Celebrate Assertive Behaviors:** Celebrate assertive behaviors and successes, recognizing the courage

and self-respect it takes to assert yourself effectively.

Guidance: Use assertiveness training exercises to develop effective communication skills and assert yourself confidently in various situations. Focus on identifying your rights, practicing assertive communication, role-playing scenarios, setting boundaries, using assertive body language, practicing self-validation, handling criticism assertively, and celebrating assertive behaviors.

Therapist Tips:

- Encourage clients to practice assertive communication regularly to build confidence and self-esteem.
- Remind clients that assertiveness is about expressing their needs and boundaries while respecting the rights and boundaries of others.
- Offer guidance and support as clients navigate assertiveness training exercises, providing validation and encouragement of their efforts to communicate assertively and advocate for themselves effectively.

Positive Affirmations

Description: This worksheet introduces positive affirmations to promote self-esteem, self-confidence, and positive self-talk.

Time: Set aside 15-20 minutes for this activity.

Activities:

1. **Identify Positive Affirmations:** Identify positive affirmations that resonate with you and reflect your strengths, values, and aspirations.

2. **Write Affirmations:** Write down your positive affirmations on paper or in a journal, using affirmative language and personalizing each affirmation to fit your unique experiences and goals.

3. **Repeat Affirmations:** Repeat your positive affirmations aloud or silently to yourself regularly, such as in the morning, throughout the day, or before challenging situations.

4. **Visualize Success:** Visualize yourself embodying the qualities and characteristics described in your affirmations, imagining yourself succeeding and achieving your goals.

5. **Challenge Negative Thoughts:** Use positive affirmations to challenge and replace negative thoughts and self-doubt with empowering and uplifting statements.

6. **Create Affirmation Cards:** Create affirmation cards or posters containing your positive affirmations and place them in visible locations as reminders of your strengths and potential.

7. **Practice Gratitude:** Practice gratitude by incorporating statements of gratitude and appreciation into your positive affirmations, fostering a positive mindset and outlook on life.

8. **Celebrate Progress:** Celebrate your progress and accomplishments, recognizing the positive changes and growth that come from practicing positive affirmations regularly.

Guidance: Use positive affirmations to cultivate self-esteem, self-confidence, and positive self-talk, fostering a more optimistic and empowering mindset. Focus on identifying positive affirmations, writing affirmations, repeating affirmations, visualizing success, challenging negative thoughts, creating affirmation cards, practicing gratitude, and celebrating progress.

Therapist Tips:

- Encourage clients to choose affirmations that resonate with them personally and reflect their goals and values.
- Remind clients that positive affirmations are most effective when practiced regularly and consistently over time.
- Offer guidance and support as clients incorporate positive affirmations into their daily routine, providing validation and encouragement of their efforts to cultivate self-esteem and self-confidence through positive self-talk.

Gratitude Journaling

Description: This worksheet introduces gratitude journaling as a practice to cultivate appreciation and positivity.

Time: Allocate 15-20 minutes for this activity.

Activities:

1. **Reflect on Blessings:** Reflect on the blessings, big or small, that you are grateful for in your life, such as relationships, experiences, opportunities, or personal qualities.
2. **Write in Journal:** Write in your gratitude journal daily, noting down three to five things you are thankful for each day, focusing on specific details and feelings associated with each blessing.
3. **Express Appreciation:** Express appreciation for the people in your life by writing thank-you notes or messages to show gratitude for their kindness, support, or presence.
4. **Practice Mindfulness:** Practice mindfulness as you journal, fully immersing yourself in the present moment and savoring the experiences and blessings you are grateful for.
5. **Reflect on Growth:** Reflect on the personal growth and lessons learned from challenging experiences or setbacks, finding gratitude for the opportunities they provide for learning and growth.

6. **Create Gratitude Rituals:** Create gratitude rituals or practices, such as saying grace before meals or taking a moment of reflection before bed, to integrate gratitude into your daily routine.
7. **Count Your Blessings:** Count your blessings regularly, acknowledging and appreciating the abundance and richness of your life, even in the midst of difficulties.
8. **Share Gratitude:** Share your gratitude with others by expressing appreciation directly or through acts of kindness and generosity, spreading positivity and goodwill.

Guidance: Use gratitude journaling as a practice to foster appreciation, positivity, and mindfulness in your daily life. Focus on reflecting on blessings, writing in your journal, expressing appreciation, practicing mindfulness, reflecting on growth, creating gratitude rituals, counting your blessings, and sharing gratitude with others.

Therapist Tips:

- Encourage clients to make gratitude journaling a regular habit by setting aside time each day to reflect on their blessings.
- Remind clients that gratitude journaling is a powerful tool for shifting focus from what is lacking to what is present and meaningful in their lives.
- Offer guidance and support as clients explore gratitude journaling, providing validation and

encouragement of their efforts to cultivate appreciation and positivity.

Self-Compassion Practices

Description: This worksheet introduces self-compassion practices to promote kindness, understanding, and acceptance towards oneself.

Time: Set aside 20-30 minutes for this activity.

Activities:

1. **Practice Self-Kindness:** Practice self-kindness by treating yourself with the same care, compassion, and empathy that you would offer to a friend in need.
2. **Cultivate Self-Understanding:** Cultivate self-understanding by acknowledging and accepting your thoughts, feelings, and experiences without judgment or criticism.
3. **Offer Self-Compassionate Statements:** Offer self-compassionate statements to yourself in moments of difficulty or distress, such as "It's okay to struggle; I am here for myself," or "May I be kind to myself in this moment."
4. **Write a Self-Compassion Letter:** Write a self-compassion letter to yourself, expressing understanding, kindness, and support towards yourself as you would to a dear friend facing similar challenges.

5. **Practice Mindfulness:** Practice mindfulness by bringing non-judgmental awareness to your thoughts, feelings, and sensations, allowing yourself to experience them without resistance or avoidance.
6. **Engage in Self-Care:** Engage in self-care activities that nurture your physical, emotional, and spiritual well-being, prioritizing your needs and replenishing your energy.
7. **Challenge Self-Criticism:** Challenge self-critical thoughts and beliefs by questioning their validity and considering alternative perspectives with kindness and curiosity.
8. **Create a Self-Compassion Mantra:** Create a self-compassion mantra or affirmation to repeat to yourself in challenging moments, such as "I am worthy of love and acceptance just as I am."

Guidance: Use self-compassion practices to cultivate kindness, understanding, and acceptance towards yourself, promoting emotional resilience and well-being. Focus on practicing self-kindness, cultivating self-understanding, offering self-compassionate statements, writing a self-compassion letter, practicing mindfulness, engaging in self-care, challenging self-criticism, and creating a self-compassion mantra.

Therapist Tips:

- Encourage clients to practice self-compassion regularly as a way to build resilience and foster emotional well-being.
- Remind clients that self-compassion is not about self-indulgence or self-pity, but rather about treating oneself with the same care and kindness as one would a friend in need.
- Offer guidance and support as clients explore self-compassion practices, providing validation and encouragement of their efforts to cultivate kindness and acceptance towards themselves.

Grounding Techniques

Description: This worksheet introduces grounding techniques to help individuals stay present and manage overwhelming emotions or anxiety.

Time: Allocate 15-20 minutes for this activity.

Activities:

1. **5-4-3-2-1 Technique:** Engage your senses by identifying and naming five things you can see, four things you can touch, three things you can hear, two things you can smell, and one thing you can taste.
2. **Square Breathing:** Practice square breathing by inhaling for a count of four, holding for a count of four, exhaling for a count of four, and holding for a count of four, repeating the cycle several times.

3. **Grounding Objects:** Carry a grounding object with you, such as a small stone or keychain, and use it as a tactile reminder to stay present and connected to the here and now.
4. **Mindful Walking:** Practice mindful walking by focusing on the sensation of each step, the movement of your body, and the contact of your feet with the ground as you walk slowly and deliberately.
5. **Body Scan Meditation:** Practice body scan meditation by systematically scanning your body from head to toe, noticing any areas of tension or discomfort and releasing them with each breath.
6. **Affirmations:** Use grounding affirmations to remind yourself that you are safe, present, and capable of coping with whatever challenges arise in the moment.
7. **Nature Connection:** Connect with nature by spending time outdoors, observing the sights, sounds, and sensations of the natural world, and grounding yourself in the beauty and tranquility of your surroundings.
8. **Breathing with Visualization:** Practice breathing with visualization by imagining yourself inhaling calm and peaceful energy and exhaling tension and stress with each breath.

Guidance: Use grounding techniques to stay present, calm, and centered during moments of distress or overwhelm. Focus on engaging your senses, practicing breathing exercises, using grounding objects, practicing mindfulness, using affirmations, connecting with nature, and breathing with visualization.

Therapist Tips:

- Encourage clients to explore different grounding techniques to find what works best for them in different situations.
- Remind clients that grounding techniques are helpful tools for managing overwhelming emotions or anxiety and can be used anywhere, anytime.
- Offer guidance and support as clients practice grounding techniques, providing validation and encouragement of their efforts to stay present and cope with distress effectively.

Emotional Regulation Strategies

Description: This worksheet introduces emotional regulation strategies to help individuals understand and manage their emotions effectively.

Time: Set aside 20-30 minutes for this activity.

Activities:

1. **Identify Triggers:** Identify common triggers or situations that provoke strong emotional reactions, such as stress, conflict, or fatigue.
2. **Practice Self-Awareness:** Practice self-awareness by recognizing and labeling your emotions as they

arise, acknowledging their intensity and impact on your thoughts and behavior.

3. **Use Coping Skills:** Use coping skills to manage overwhelming emotions, such as deep breathing, progressive muscle relaxation, mindfulness meditation, or engaging in enjoyable activities.

4. **Cognitive Restructuring:** Practice cognitive restructuring by challenging and reframing negative or irrational thoughts that contribute to intense emotions, replacing them with more balanced and realistic perspectives.

5. **Express Emotions:** Express your emotions in healthy ways, such as journaling, talking to a trusted friend or therapist, or engaging in creative outlets like art or music.

6. **Set Boundaries:** Set boundaries in relationships and interactions to protect your emotional well-being, assertively communicating your needs and limits to others.

7. **Seek Support:** Seek support from others when needed, reaching out to friends, family, or professionals for validation, empathy, and guidance in managing emotions.

8. **Practice Self-Care:** Prioritize self-care activities that nurture your physical, emotional, and spiritual well-being, replenishing your energy and resilience.

Guidance: Use emotional regulation strategies to understand and manage your emotions effectively, promoting emotional well-being and resilience. Focus on identifying triggers, practicing self-awareness, using coping skills, cognitive restructuring, expressing emotions, setting boundaries, seeking support, and practicing self-care.

Therapist Tips:

- Encourage clients to practice emotional regulation strategies regularly to build resilience and cope with difficult emotions.
- Remind clients that it's okay to experience a wide range of emotions and that they have the ability to manage their emotions effectively with practice and support.
- Offer guidance and support as clients explore emotional regulation strategies, providing validation and encouragement of their efforts to understand and cope with their emotions effectively.

Section 4: Cognitive-Behavioral Techniques

In this section, individuals will find a range of worksheets and exercises designed to help them address underlying cognitive and behavioral factors contributing to their substance abuse.

Challenging Negative Thoughts

Description: This worksheet guides individuals in identifying and challenging negative thoughts and irrational beliefs related to substance use.

Time: Allocate 20-30 minutes for this activity.

Activities:

1. **Identify Negative Thoughts:** Identify negative thoughts or beliefs related to substance use, such as "I can't cope without drugs" or "I'm worthless without alcohol."
2. **Evaluate Evidence:** Evaluate the evidence supporting these negative thoughts, considering whether they are based on facts or distorted perceptions.
3. **Challenge Negative Thoughts:** Challenge negative thoughts by questioning their accuracy and exploring alternative, more balanced perspectives.
4. **Generate Counterarguments:** Generate counterarguments or alternative thoughts that contradict the negative beliefs, focusing on evidence-based reasoning and realistic expectations.
5. **Reframe Thoughts:** Reframe negative thoughts into more adaptive and empowering statements, emphasizing resilience, self-efficacy, and growth.
6. **Practice Affirmations:** Practice affirmations or positive self-talk to reinforce the revised, more

positive beliefs, fostering a sense of confidence and self-worth.

7. **Track Progress:** Track progress by monitoring changes in thought patterns and emotional responses over time, celebrating successes and addressing challenges as they arise.

Guidance: Use this worksheet to challenge and reframe negative thoughts and beliefs related to substance use, promoting healthier thinking patterns and attitudes towards recovery. Focus on identifying negative thoughts, evaluating evidence, challenging thoughts, generating counterarguments, reframing thoughts, practicing affirmations, and tracking progress.

Therapist Tips:

- Encourage clients to approach negative thoughts with curiosity and openness, exploring their origins and validity.
- Remind clients that challenging negative thoughts is a skill that improves with practice and persistence.
- Offer guidance and support as clients work through challenging negative thoughts, providing validation and encouragement of their efforts to cultivate more adaptive thinking patterns.

Thought Records

Description: This worksheet provides a template for recording and analyzing thoughts and emotions associated with cravings and substance use.

Time: Set aside 20-30 minutes for this activity.

Activities:

1. **Identify Triggering Situation:** Identify the triggering situation or event that led to the craving or urge to use substances.
2. **Record Thoughts:** Record the thoughts and beliefs that accompanied the craving, paying attention to any irrational or distorted thinking patterns.
3. **Rate Intensity:** Rate the intensity of the craving or urge on a scale from 1 to 10, indicating its strength and immediacy.
4. **Challenge Thoughts:** Challenge the accuracy and validity of the thoughts recorded, considering alternative perspectives and evidence-based reasoning.
5. **Generate Alternative Thoughts:** Generate alternative, more balanced thoughts that contradict the negative or irrational beliefs, promoting healthier coping strategies.
6. **Reassess Intensity:** Reassess the intensity of the craving after challenging and reframing the thoughts, noting any changes in its strength or urgency.

7. **Develop Coping Strategies:** Develop coping strategies or action plans to manage the craving effectively, drawing on healthier alternatives to substance use.

8. **Reflect on Learning:** Reflect on the insights gained from completing the thought record, identifying patterns, triggers, and effective coping strategies for future use.

Guidance: Use this worksheet to record and analyze thoughts and emotions associated with cravings and substance use, fostering self-awareness and developing effective coping strategies. Focus on identifying triggering situations, recording thoughts, rating intensity, challenging thoughts, generating alternatives, reassessing intensity, developing coping strategies, and reflecting on learning.

Therapist Tips:

- Encourage clients to use thought records as a tool for increasing self-awareness and developing healthier responses to cravings.
- Remind clients that thought records are most effective when completed in the moment, capturing thoughts and emotions as they occur.
- Offer guidance and support as clients work through thought records, providing validation and encouragement of their efforts to manage cravings and promote recovery.

Cognitive Restructuring

Description: This worksheet provides exercises to reframe negative thought patterns and develop more positive thinking habits related to substance use.

Time: Allocate 20-30 minutes for this activity.

Activities:

1. **Identify Negative Thoughts:** Identify recurring negative thoughts or beliefs related to substance use, such as "I can't have fun without drinking" or "Using drugs is the only way to cope with stress."
2. **Challenge Distorted Thinking:** Challenge distorted thinking by examining the evidence for and against the negative beliefs, considering alternative explanations and viewpoints.
3. **Reframe Negative Thoughts:** Reframe negative thoughts into more balanced and realistic statements, emphasizing resilience, coping skills, and personal strengths.
4. **Practice Positive Affirmations:** Practice positive affirmations or self-statements to reinforce the revised, more positive beliefs, fostering self-compassion and self-empowerment.
5. **Visualize Success:** Visualize success and positive outcomes related to sobriety, imagining yourself overcoming challenges and living a fulfilling, substance-free life.

6. **Develop Coping Strategies:** Develop coping strategies or action plans to manage triggers and cravings effectively, drawing on the new, more adaptive beliefs and attitudes.

7. **Challenge Automatic Thoughts:** Challenge automatic thoughts related to substance use in the moment, using cognitive restructuring techniques to shift perspective and reduce impulsivity.

Guidance: Use this worksheet to reframe negative thought patterns and cultivate more positive thinking habits in relation to substance use, promoting resilience and recovery. Focus on identifying negative thoughts, challenging distorted thinking, reframing thoughts, practicing positive affirmations, visualizing success, developing coping strategies, and challenging automatic thoughts.

Therapist Tips:

- Encourage clients to approach cognitive restructuring with openness and curiosity, exploring the impact of their thoughts on their emotions and behaviors.
- Remind clients that cognitive restructuring is a skill that requires practice and patience, but can lead to profound shifts in perspective and behavior.
- Offer guidance and support as clients work through cognitive restructuring exercises, providing validation and encouragement of their efforts to

cultivate more adaptive thinking patterns and promote recovery.

Positive Self-Talk

Description: This worksheet introduces positive self-talk techniques to promote self-compassion, self-empowerment, and resilience in recovery from substance abuse.

Time: Set aside 15-20 minutes for this activity.

Activities:

1. **Identify Negative Self-Talk:** Identify common negative self-talk patterns or inner critics related to substance use, such as self-criticism, self-doubt, or self-blame.
2. **Challenge Negative Self-Talk:** Challenge negative self-talk by questioning its accuracy and validity, considering alternative perspectives and evidence-based reasoning.
3. **Replace with Positive Affirmations:** Replace negative self-talk with positive affirmations or self-statements that promote self-compassion, self-empowerment, and resilience.
4. **Practice Daily Affirmations:** Practice daily affirmations by repeating positive self-talk statements regularly, incorporating them into your daily routine and self-care practices.

5. **Visualize Success:** Visualize success and positive outcomes related to sobriety, imagining yourself overcoming challenges and achieving your goals with confidence and determination.

6. **Create a Self-Encouragement Mantra:** Create a self-encouragement mantra or affirmation to repeat to yourself in moments of doubt or difficulty, reinforcing your resilience and commitment to recovery.

7. **Reflect on Progress:** Reflect on your progress in replacing negative self-talk with positive affirmations, celebrating successes and acknowledging challenges as opportunities for growth and learning.

Guidance: Use this worksheet to cultivate positive self-talk and promote self-compassion, self-empowerment, and resilience in recovery from substance abuse. Focus on identifying negative self-talk, challenging it, replacing it with positive affirmations, practicing daily affirmations, visualizing success, creating a self-encouragement mantra, and reflecting on progress.

Therapist Tips:

- Encourage clients to practice positive self-talk regularly as a way to build self-compassion and resilience in recovery.
- Remind clients that positive self-talk is a powerful tool for shifting perspective and fostering a sense of empowerment and self-worth.

- Offer guidance and support as clients explore positive self-talk techniques, providing validation and encouragement of their efforts to cultivate a more supportive inner dialogue.

Behavioral Activation

Description: This worksheet introduces behavioral activation techniques to increase engagement in positive, rewarding activities and decrease reliance on substance use.

Time: Allocate 20-30 minutes for this activity.

Activities:

1. **Identify Pleasant Activities:** Identify activities that bring joy, satisfaction, or fulfillment, such as hobbies, socializing, exercise, or creative pursuits.
2. **Create Activity Schedule:** Create a weekly activity schedule, incorporating a variety of pleasant activities to balance work, leisure, and self-care.
3. **Set SMART Goals:** Set SMART (Specific, Measurable, Achievable, Relevant, Time-bound) goals for each activity, clarifying what you hope to accomplish and how you will measure success.
4. **Schedule Activities:** Schedule specific times for each activity in your weekly calendar, prioritizing self-care and leisure activities alongside work or other responsibilities.
5. **Monitor Progress:** Monitor your progress in engaging in planned activities, tracking adherence

to your schedule and noting any barriers or challenges that arise.

6. **Adapt and Adjust:** Adapt your activity schedule as needed based on feedback and experiences, being flexible and open to trying new activities or adjusting goals.

7. **Reflect on Enjoyment:** Reflect on your enjoyment and satisfaction after engaging in each activity, identifying which activities are most meaningful and rewarding for you.

8. **Practice Self-Compassion:** Practice self-compassion and non-judgmental acceptance of yourself, acknowledging efforts and progress rather than focusing on perceived shortcomings or setbacks.

Guidance: Use this worksheet to increase engagement in positive, rewarding activities as a way to reduce reliance on substance use and enhance overall well-being. Focus on identifying pleasant activities, creating an activity schedule, setting SMART goals, scheduling activities, monitoring progress, adapting and adjusting, reflecting on enjoyment, and practicing self-compassion.

Therapist Tips:

- Encourage clients to start small and gradually increase the frequency and variety of activities over time.
- Remind clients that behavioral activation is a key component of maintaining sobriety and promoting emotional well-being.

- Offer guidance and support as clients explore behavioral activation techniques, providing validation and encouragement of their efforts to increase engagement in positive activities and decrease reliance on substances.

Role-Playing and Rehearsal

Description: This worksheet introduces role-playing and rehearsal techniques to practice assertive communication skills and coping strategies in challenging situations related to substance use.

Time: Set aside 20-30 minutes for this activity.

Activities:

1. **Identify Challenging Situations:** Identify challenging situations or scenarios where assertive communication and coping skills may be beneficial, such as social gatherings or encounters with triggers.
2. **Role-Play Scenarios:** Role-play each challenging scenario with a trusted friend, family member, or therapist, taking turns playing different roles and practicing assertive communication techniques.
3. **Rehearse Responses:** Rehearse assertive responses and coping strategies for each scenario, focusing on clear communication, boundary-setting, and problem-solving skills.
4. **Receive Feedback:** Receive feedback from your role-playing partner or therapist on your

communication style, assertiveness, and effectiveness of coping strategies.

5. **Reflect on Learning:** Reflect on the experience of role-playing and rehearsal, identifying strengths, areas for improvement, and insights gained for future use.

6. **Generalize Skills:** Generalize assertive communication and coping skills from role-playing scenarios to real-life situations, applying what you've learned in challenging encounters with substance-related triggers or stressors.

Guidance: Use this worksheet to practice assertive communication skills and coping strategies in challenging situations related to substance use, promoting confidence and effectiveness in managing triggers and cravings. Focus on identifying challenging situations, role-playing scenarios, rehearsing responses, receiving feedback, reflecting on learning, and generalizing skills.

Therapist Tips:

- Encourage clients to approach role-playing and rehearsal with an open mind and willingness to experiment with different communication styles and coping strategies.
- Remind clients that assertive communication is a skill that can be learned and improved with practice over time.
- Offer guidance and support as clients practice role-playing and rehearsal techniques, providing

validation and encouragement of their efforts to develop assertiveness and coping skills in challenging situations.

Mindfulness Meditation

Description: This worksheet introduces mindfulness meditation techniques to cultivate present-moment awareness and reduce reactivity to cravings and triggers related to substance use.

Time: Allocate 20-30 minutes for this activity.

Activities:

1. **Settle into a Comfortable Position:** Find a comfortable seated or lying position, ensuring that your body is relaxed and supported.
2. **Focus on the Breath:** Bring your attention to the sensations of your breath, noticing the rise and fall of your chest or abdomen with each inhale and exhale.
3. **Notice Thoughts and Sensations:** Notice any thoughts, emotions, or sensations that arise during meditation, observing them with curiosity and non-judgment.
4. **Return to the Breath:** Whenever you notice your mind wandering or becoming caught up in thoughts, gently redirect your focus back to the breath.
5. **Expand Awareness:** Expand your awareness to include other sensations in the body, such as the

feeling of contact with the ground or the sensation of air on your skin.

6. **Practice Acceptance:** Practice acceptance of whatever arises during meditation, allowing thoughts and emotions to come and go without attachment or resistance.

7. **Cultivate Compassion:** Cultivate compassion for yourself and others during meditation, extending kindness and understanding to all aspects of your experience.

8. **End with Gratitude:** End your meditation practice with a sense of gratitude for the opportunity to cultivate mindfulness and presence in your life.

Guidance: Use this worksheet to practice mindfulness meditation as a way to cultivate present-moment awareness and reduce reactivity to cravings and triggers related to substance use. Focus on settling into a comfortable position, focusing on the breath, noticing thoughts and sensations, returning to the breath, expanding awareness, practicing acceptance, cultivating compassion, and ending with gratitude.

Therapist Tips:

- Encourage clients to approach mindfulness meditation with an attitude of openness, curiosity, and non-judgment.
- Remind clients that mindfulness is a skill that develops with practice over time, and that consistency is more important than perfection.

- Offer guidance and support as clients explore mindfulness meditation techniques, providing validation and encouragement of their efforts to cultivate present-moment awareness and reduce reactivity to cravings and triggers.

Grounding Techniques

Description: This worksheet introduces grounding techniques to help individuals stay connected to the present moment and manage distressing thoughts and emotions related to substance use.

Time: Set aside 15-20 minutes for this activity.

Activities:

1. **Five Senses Exercise:** Engage your five senses by identifying and focusing on five things you can see, four things you can touch, three things you can hear, two things you can smell, and one thing you can taste.
2. **Deep Breathing:** Practice deep breathing exercises to promote relaxation and reduce physiological arousal, taking slow, deep breaths in through the nose and out through the mouth.
3. **Progressive Muscle Relaxation:** Engage in progressive muscle relaxation by tensing and then relaxing each muscle group in your body, starting from your toes and working your way up to your head.

4. **Visual Imagery:** Use visual imagery to create a mental image of a safe, calming place or situation, imagining yourself in this space and focusing on the details.
5. **Positive Affirmations:** Repeat positive affirmations or self-statements to yourself, affirming your ability to cope with challenges and manage distress effectively.
6. **Grounding Objects:** Hold onto a grounding object such as a smooth stone, piece of fabric, or stress ball, focusing on its texture, weight, and temperature as a way to anchor yourself in the present moment.
7. **Mindful Movement:** Engage in mindful movement practices such as walking, stretching, or yoga, paying attention to the sensations in your body as you move.

Guidance: Use this worksheet to practice grounding techniques as a way to stay connected to the present moment and manage distressing thoughts and emotions related to substance use. Focus on engaging the five senses, deep breathing, progressive muscle relaxation, visual imagery, positive affirmations, grounding objects, and mindful movement.

Therapist Tips:

*   Encourage clients to experiment with different grounding techniques to find what works best for them in different situations.

- Remind clients that grounding techniques can be used anytime, anywhere, as a way to manage distress and promote emotional regulation.
- Offer guidance and support as clients practice grounding techniques, providing validation and encouragement of their efforts to stay connected to the present moment and manage distress effectively.

Distress Tolerance Strategies

Description: This worksheet introduces distress tolerance strategies to help individuals cope with intense emotions and urges related to substance use without resorting to harmful behaviors.

Time: Allocate 20-30 minutes for this activity.

Activities:

1. **STOP Technique:** Use the STOP technique to pause and take a break when experiencing intense emotions or urges related to substance use. Stop what you're doing, take a few deep breaths, observe your thoughts and feelings, and proceed mindfully.
2. **Self-Soothing Activities:** Engage in self-soothing activities that promote relaxation and comfort, such as taking a warm bath, listening to soothing music, or cuddling with a pet.
3. **Distraction Techniques:** Distract yourself from distressing thoughts or emotions by focusing your

attention on a neutral or engaging activity, such as reading a book, watching a funny movie, or going for a walk.

4. **Thought Defusion:** Practice thought defusion techniques to distance yourself from distressing thoughts and reduce their impact on your emotions and behavior, such as imagining thoughts as passing clouds or leaves on a stream.

5. **Urge Surfing:** Practice urge surfing by riding out intense cravings or urges related to substance use without acting on them, observing the rise and fall of the urge like a wave until it naturally dissipates.

6. **Crisis Survival Skills:** Develop a crisis survival plan that includes specific coping strategies and support resources to use in moments of intense distress or crisis related to substance use.

Guidance: Use this worksheet to explore distress tolerance strategies as a way to cope with intense emotions and urges related to substance use. Focus on using the STOP technique, engaging in self-soothing activities, practicing distraction techniques, using thought defusion, practicing urge surfing, and developing a crisis survival plan.

Therapist Tips:

- Encourage clients to practice distress tolerance strategies regularly, even during times of low distress, to build resilience and preparedness for challenging situations.

- Remind clients that distress tolerance is a skill that can be developed and strengthened with practice over time.
- Offer guidance and support as clients explore distress tolerance techniques, providing validation and encouragement of their efforts to cope with intense emotions and urges related to substance use.

Acceptance and Commitment Therapy (ACT) Techniques

Description: This worksheet introduces acceptance and commitment therapy (ACT) techniques to help individuals accept difficult thoughts and emotions related to substance use and commit to values-based actions.

Time: Set aside 20-30 minutes for this activity.

Activities:

1. **Mindfulness of Thoughts and Emotions:** Practice mindfulness of thoughts and emotions by observing them with curiosity and non-judgment, acknowledging their presence without trying to change or suppress them.
2. **Values Clarification:** Clarify your values and priorities in life, identifying what truly matters to you and what you want to stand for.
3. **Cognitive Defusion:** Practice cognitive defusion techniques to distance yourself from unhelpful

thoughts and reduce their impact on your behavior, such as imagining thoughts as passing clouds or leaves on a stream.

4. **Committed Action:** Identify concrete actions aligned with your values and commit to taking steps toward these goals, even in the face of discomfort or uncertainty.

5. **Expansion Exercises:** Engage in expansion exercises to broaden your awareness and embrace the full range of human experience, including both joy and pain.

6. **Self-Compassion:** Cultivate self-compassion and acceptance toward yourself, acknowledging your struggles and imperfections with kindness and understanding.

Guidance: Use this worksheet to explore acceptance and commitment therapy (ACT) techniques as a way to accept difficult thoughts and emotions related to substance use and commit to values-based actions. Focus on practicing mindfulness of thoughts and emotions, clarifying values, using cognitive defusion, committing to action, engaging in expansion exercises, and cultivating self-compassion.

Therapist Tips:

- Encourage clients to approach acceptance and commitment therapy (ACT) techniques with openness and curiosity, exploring the role of acceptance and values in their recovery journey.

- Remind clients that acceptance does not mean resignation or approval of harmful behaviors, but rather a willingness to acknowledge reality as it is and take steps toward meaningful change.
- Offer guidance and support as clients explore ACT techniques, providing validation and encouragement of their efforts to accept difficult thoughts and emotions related to substance use and commit to values-based actions.

Emotional Regulation Strategies

Description: This worksheet introduces emotional regulation strategies to help individuals identify, understand, and manage intense emotions related to substance use.

Time: Allocate 20-30 minutes for this activity.

Activities:

1. **Emotion Identification:** Practice identifying and labeling emotions accurately, using an emotion wheel or list of emotion words to expand your emotional vocabulary.
2. **Emotion Validation:** Validate your emotions by acknowledging their presence and understanding their underlying causes and triggers, without judgment or criticism.
3. **Emotion Regulation Techniques:** Use emotion regulation techniques such as deep breathing, progressive muscle relaxation, or grounding

exercises to reduce physiological arousal and promote emotional balance.

4. **Cognitive Reappraisal:** Reappraise distressing situations or events from a more balanced or neutral perspective, challenging unhelpful thoughts and beliefs that contribute to emotional distress.

5. **Expressive Writing:** Engage in expressive writing exercises to process and release intense emotions, writing freely and uncensored about your thoughts and feelings related to substance use.

6. **Problem-Solving Skills:** Develop problem-solving skills to address underlying issues or stressors that contribute to emotional distress, brainstorming solutions and taking action to address them.

7. **Seeking Social Support:** Reach out to trusted friends, family members, or support groups for validation, empathy, and practical assistance in coping with intense emotions related to substance use.

Guidance: Use this worksheet to explore emotional regulation strategies as a way to identify, understand, and manage intense emotions related to substance use. Focus on emotion identification, validation, regulation techniques, cognitive reappraisal, expressive writing, problem-solving skills, and seeking social support.

Therapist Tips:

- Encourage clients to practice emotional regulation strategies regularly, even during times of low distress, to build resilience and emotional well-being.

- Remind clients that emotions are a natural and valid part of the human experience, and that it's okay to feel and express them.
- Offer guidance and support as clients explore emotional regulation techniques, providing validation and encouragement of their efforts to identify, understand, and manage intense emotions related to substance use.

Section 5: Relapse Prevention Strategies

Section 5 serves as a valuable resource for individuals to proactively manage and reduce the risk of relapse, empowering them to maintain their sobriety and continue their journey of recovery with confidence and resilience. Each worksheet in this section provides clear instructions and guidance on how to implement relapse prevention strategies effectively. Therapist tips may also be included to offer additional insights and support.

Warning Signs of Relapse

Description: This worksheet helps individuals recognize early signs of relapse and intervene effectively to prevent a return to substance use.

Time: Allocate 15-20 minutes for this activity.

Activities:

1. **Identify Personal Triggers:** Reflect on past experiences and identify personal triggers or warning signs that have preceded relapse in the past.
2. **Recognize Early Warning Signs:** Recognize early warning signs of relapse, such as increased cravings, mood swings, withdrawal symptoms, or changes in behavior.
3. **Monitor Physical and Emotional Symptoms:** Monitor physical and emotional symptoms regularly to detect any changes that may indicate increased vulnerability to relapse.
4. **Create an Early Warning System:** Develop a personalized early warning system to track and respond to warning signs effectively, such as keeping a daily journal or using a smartphone app to monitor mood and cravings.
5. **Reach Out for Support:** Reach out to trusted friends, family members, or support groups for guidance and support when early warning signs of relapse are identified.

Guidance: Use this worksheet to recognize early signs of relapse and intervene effectively to prevent a return to substance use. Focus on identifying personal triggers, recognizing early warning signs, monitoring physical and emotional symptoms, creating an early warning system, and reaching out for support.

Therapist Tips:

- Encourage clients to be proactive in monitoring their own warning signs of relapse and taking action to address them promptly.
- Remind clients that relapse prevention is an ongoing process that requires vigilance and self-awareness.
- Offer guidance and support as clients explore warning signs of relapse, providing validation and encouragement of their efforts to maintain sobriety and prevent relapse.

Developing a Relapse Prevention Plan

Description: This worksheet provides a step-by-step guide to creating a personalized plan to prevent relapse and maintain sobriety.

Time: Set aside 30-45 minutes for this activity.

Activities:

1. **Identify Triggers and High-Risk Situations:** Identify personal triggers and high-risk situations that may

increase vulnerability to relapse, such as stress, negative emotions, or social pressures.

2. **List Coping Strategies:** Create a list of coping strategies and techniques that have been effective in managing cravings and urges to use substances in the past.

3. **Develop an Action Plan:** Develop a step-by-step action plan outlining specific steps to take when confronted with triggers or cravings, including alternative activities, coping skills, and support resources.

4. **Establish Support Network:** Establish a support network of trusted individuals who can provide guidance, encouragement, and accountability in maintaining sobriety.

5. **Review and Revise Plan:** Review and revise the relapse prevention plan regularly to adapt to changing circumstances, experiences, and needs.

Guidance: Use this worksheet to develop a relapse prevention plan tailored to individual needs and circumstances. Focus on identifying triggers and high-risk situations, listing coping strategies, developing an action plan, establishing a support network, and reviewing and revising the plan regularly.

Therapist Tips:

- Encourage clients to be thorough and specific in developing their relapse prevention plan, considering a wide range of potential triggers and coping strategies.

- Remind clients that a relapse prevention plan is a dynamic document that can be revised and updated as needed over time.
- Offer guidance and support as clients develop their relapse prevention plan, providing validation and encouragement of their efforts to maintain sobriety and prevent relapse.

Creating Emergency Coping Strategies

Description: This worksheet helps individuals prepare for unexpected triggers or cravings by developing emergency coping strategies.

Time: Allocate 15-20 minutes for this activity.

Activities:

1. **Identify Potential Triggers:** Reflect on past experiences and identify potential triggers or situations that may lead to cravings or urges to use substances unexpectedly.
2. **Brainstorm Coping Strategies:** Brainstorm a list of coping strategies and techniques that can be used in emergency situations to manage cravings or urges effectively.
3. **Select Effective Coping Techniques:** Select the most effective coping techniques from the list, considering factors such as accessibility, ease of

implementation, and previous success in managing cravings.

4. **Practice Coping Skills:** Practice implementing the selected coping techniques in simulated or imagined emergency situations to build confidence and familiarity with their use.

5. **Create a Coping Plan:** Develop a personalized coping plan outlining specific steps to take when faced with unexpected triggers or cravings, including alternative activities, coping skills, and support resources.

Guidance: Use this worksheet to create emergency coping strategies for managing unexpected triggers or cravings related to substance use. Focus on identifying potential triggers, brainstorming coping strategies, selecting effective techniques, practicing coping skills, and creating a coping plan.

Therapist Tips:

- Encourage clients to be proactive in preparing for unexpected triggers or cravings by developing a range of coping strategies that can be used in emergency situations.
- Remind clients that practice is essential for building confidence and competence in using coping skills effectively.
- Offer guidance and support as clients create their emergency coping strategies, providing validation

and encouragement of their efforts to maintain sobriety and manage cravings.

Post-Relapse Reflection

Description: This worksheet provides a structured framework for reflecting on triggers and coping strategies following a relapse.

Time: Set aside 20-30 minutes for this activity.

Activities:

1. **Review Relapse Experience:** Reflect on the circumstances and events leading up to the relapse, including triggers, high-risk situations, and emotional states.
2. **Identify Warning Signs:** Identify warning signs and early indicators of relapse that may have been overlooked or ignored in the lead-up to the relapse.
3. **Assess Coping Strategies:** Evaluate the effectiveness of coping strategies and techniques used to manage cravings and urges leading up to the relapse.
4. **Identify Learning Points:** Identify key learning points and insights gained from the relapse experience, including strengths and areas for growth.
5. **Develop Relapse Prevention Plan:** Use insights gained from the reflection process to revise and strengthen the relapse prevention plan,

incorporating new coping strategies and support resources.

Guidance: Use this worksheet to reflect on triggers and coping strategies following a relapse, with the goal of learning from the experience and strengthening relapse prevention efforts. Focus on reviewing the relapse experience, identifying warning signs, assessing coping strategies, identifying learning points, and developing a relapse prevention plan.

Therapist Tips:

- Encourage clients to approach post-relapse reflection with curiosity and self-compassion, focusing on learning and growth rather than self-criticism.
- Remind clients that relapse is a common and often unavoidable part of the recovery process, and that it can provide valuable insights for strengthening relapse prevention efforts.
- Offer guidance and support as clients engage in post-relapse reflection, providing validation and encouragement of their efforts to learn from their experiences and maintain sobriety.

Identifying High-Risk Situations

Description: This worksheet helps individuals identify high-risk situations that may increase the likelihood of relapse.

Time: Allocate 15-20 minutes for this activity.

Activities:

1. **Reflect on Past Experiences:** Reflect on past instances of substance use or relapse and identify the specific situations, emotions, people, or places that were present.
2. **Identify Triggers:** Identify triggers or cues associated with high-risk situations, such as stress, negative emotions, peer pressure, or exposure to substances.
3. **Assess Vulnerability:** Assess personal vulnerability factors that may increase susceptibility to high-risk situations, such as low self-esteem, poor coping skills, or lack of social support.
4. **Develop Coping Strategies:** Develop coping strategies and techniques to manage high-risk situations effectively, such as stress management techniques, assertiveness skills, or refusal skills.
5. **Create a High-Risk Situation Plan:** Create a personalized plan outlining steps to take when faced with high-risk situations, including alternative activities, coping skills, and support resources.

Guidance: Use this worksheet to identify high-risk situations that may increase the likelihood of relapse and develop strategies for managing them effectively. Focus on reflecting on past experiences, identifying triggers, assessing vulnerability factors, developing coping strategies, and creating a high-risk situation plan.

Therapist Tips:

- Encourage clients to approach the identification of high-risk situations with honesty and self-awareness, acknowledging areas of vulnerability and potential triggers.
- Remind clients that relapse prevention is an ongoing process that requires vigilance and proactive planning to manage high-risk situations effectively.
- Offer guidance and support as clients develop their high-risk situation plan, providing validation and encouragement of their efforts to maintain sobriety and prevent relapse.

Building Healthy Habits

Description: This worksheet helps individuals establish healthy habits and routines to support long-term recovery from substance abuse.

Time: Set aside 20-30 minutes for this activity.

Activities:

1. **Identify Areas for Improvement:** Reflect on current habits and routines related to diet, exercise, sleep,

self-care, and leisure activities, and identify areas for improvement.

2. **Set Specific Goals:** Set specific, measurable, achievable, relevant, and time-bound (SMART) goals for building healthy habits in each area identified for improvement.

3. **Develop Action Plans:** Develop action plans outlining concrete steps to achieve each SMART goal, including specific activities, timelines, and milestones.

4. **Implement Strategies:** Implement strategies for overcoming barriers and obstacles to building healthy habits, such as time management techniques, stress management strategies, or seeking support from others.

5. **Monitor Progress:** Monitor progress toward building healthy habits regularly, tracking adherence to action plans and adjusting goals as needed based on feedback and results.

Guidance: Use this worksheet to build healthy habits and routines that support long-term recovery from substance abuse. Focus on identifying areas for improvement, setting specific goals, developing action plans, implementing strategies, and monitoring progress.

Therapist Tips:

- Encourage clients to start small and focus on making gradual, sustainable changes to their habits and routines over time.

- Remind clients that building healthy habits is a process that requires patience, perseverance, and self-compassion.
- Offer guidance and support as clients develop their action plans and implement strategies for building healthy habits, providing validation and encouragement of their efforts to support their recovery journey.

Assertiveness Training

Description: This worksheet introduces assertiveness training exercises to help individuals develop assertive communication skills in various situations related to substance use.

Time: Allocate 20-30 minutes for this activity.

Activities:

1. **Understanding Assertiveness:** Define assertiveness and differentiate it from passive and aggressive communication styles, discussing the benefits of assertive communication in recovery.
2. **Identifying Assertive Responses:** Identify assertive responses to common scenarios related to substance use, such as refusing offers of substances, setting boundaries with peers, or expressing needs and preferences.
3. **Role-Playing Exercises:** Engage in role-playing exercises to practice assertive communication skills

216

in simulated or imagined situations, receiving feedback and support from peers or a therapist.

4. **Assertiveness Scripts:** Develop assertiveness scripts or statements to use in specific situations, such as saying "no" to offers of substances or expressing feelings and preferences assertively.

5. **Reflective Journaling:** Reflect on experiences of practicing assertive communication skills, noting successes, challenges, and areas for improvement.

Guidance: Use this worksheet to develop assertive communication skills in various situations related to substance use, promoting healthy boundaries and self-advocacy. Focus on understanding assertiveness, identifying assertive responses, engaging in role-playing exercises, developing assertiveness scripts, and reflecting on experiences.

Therapist Tips:

- Encourage clients to practice assertive communication skills regularly, both in therapy sessions and in real-life situations.
- Remind clients that assertiveness is a learned skill that improves with practice and feedback from others.
- Offer guidance and support as clients navigate assertiveness training exercises, providing validation and encouragement of their efforts to develop healthy communication skills in recovery.

Mindfulness Meditation

Description: This worksheet introduces mindfulness meditation as a coping strategy for managing cravings and stress associated with substance abuse.

Time: Allocate 15-20 minutes for this activity.

Activities:

1. **Understanding Mindfulness:** Define mindfulness and discuss its benefits for managing cravings, reducing stress, and promoting overall well-being in recovery.
2. **Guided Meditation:** Guide participants through a mindfulness meditation practice focused on observing sensations, thoughts, and emotions without judgment.
3. **Body Scan Exercise:** Lead participants through a body scan exercise, directing attention to different parts of the body and noticing sensations with curiosity and acceptance.
4. **Breathing Awareness:** Practice breathing awareness exercises, focusing on the sensation of the breath as it enters and leaves the body, anchoring attention in the present moment.
5. **Reflective Journaling:** Encourage participants to reflect on their experiences with mindfulness meditation, noting any insights, challenges, or benefits observed during the practice.

Guidance: Use this worksheet to introduce mindfulness meditation as a coping strategy for managing cravings and stress in recovery. Focus on understanding mindfulness, practicing guided meditation, body scan exercises, breathing awareness, and reflecting on experiences.

Therapist Tips:

- Emphasize the importance of regular mindfulness practice for cultivating awareness, self-regulation, and emotional resilience in recovery.
- Encourage participants to approach mindfulness meditation with an open mind and a non-judgmental attitude, allowing thoughts and emotions to arise and pass without attachment.
- Offer guidance and support as participants explore mindfulness meditation, providing validation and encouragement of their efforts to cultivate mindfulness in their daily lives.

Progressive Muscle Relaxation (PMR)

Description: This worksheet introduces progressive muscle relaxation (PMR) as a technique for reducing muscle tension and promoting relaxation in recovery.

Time: Set aside 15-20 minutes for this activity.

Activities:

1. **Understanding PMR:** Explain the concept of progressive muscle relaxation and its benefits for managing physical tension and stress in recovery.

2. **Guided PMR Exercise:** Guide participants through a progressive muscle relaxation exercise, systematically tensing and relaxing different muscle groups in the body.
3. **Body Awareness Scan:** Lead participants through a body awareness scan, encouraging them to notice areas of tension or discomfort and release tension with each exhalation.
4. **Breathing Techniques:** Combine PMR with deep breathing techniques, synchronizing muscle relaxation with slow, deep breaths to enhance relaxation and stress relief.
5. **Reflective Journaling:** Prompt participants to journal about their experience with PMR, noting any changes in physical tension, stress levels, or overall well-being observed during the practice.

Guidance: Use this worksheet to introduce progressive muscle relaxation (PMR) as a technique for reducing muscle tension and promoting relaxation in recovery. Focus on understanding PMR, practicing guided PMR exercises, body awareness scans, breathing techniques, and reflecting on experiences.

Therapist Tips:

- Encourage participants to practice progressive muscle relaxation regularly, incorporating it into their daily routine as a tool for managing stress and promoting relaxation.

- Remind participants to approach PMR with patience and self-compassion, allowing themselves to relax at their own pace without judgment.
- Offer guidance and support as participants explore progressive muscle relaxation, providing validation and encouragement of their efforts to cultivate relaxation in their daily lives.

Visualization Techniques

Description: This worksheet introduces visualization techniques as a strategy for managing cravings and promoting relaxation in recovery.

Time: Allocate 15-20 minutes for this activity.

Activities:

1. **Understanding Visualization:** Explain the concept of visualization and its benefits for managing cravings, reducing stress, and promoting relaxation in recovery.
2. **Guided Visualization Exercise:** Guide participants through a visualization exercise, instructing them to imagine a peaceful, calming scene or a scenario where they successfully resist cravings and maintain sobriety.
3. **Using Imagery:** Encourage participants to use vivid imagery and engage all the senses during the visualization exercise, enhancing the effectiveness of the practice.

4. **Positive Affirmations:** Incorporate positive affirmations or statements into the visualization exercise, reinforcing beliefs in one's ability to cope with cravings and maintain sobriety.
5. **Reflective Journaling:** Prompt participants to journal about their experience with visualization, noting any feelings of relaxation, empowerment, or confidence generated by the practice.

Guidance: Use this worksheet to introduce visualization techniques as a strategy for managing cravings and promoting relaxation in recovery. Focus on understanding visualization, practicing guided visualization exercises, using imagery, incorporating positive affirmations, and reflecting on experiences.

Therapist Tips:

- Encourage participants to practice visualization regularly, incorporating it into their daily routine as a tool for managing cravings and promoting relaxation.
- Remind participants to engage all the senses and create a vivid mental image during the visualization exercise, enhancing its effectiveness.
- Offer guidance and support as participants explore visualization techniques, providing validation and encouragement of their efforts to cultivate relaxation and coping skills in their daily lives

Distraction Techniques

Description: This worksheet introduces distraction techniques as a strategy for managing cravings and shifting focus away from substance use triggers.

Time: Set aside 15-20 minutes for this activity.

Activities:

1. **Understanding Distraction:** Explain the concept of distraction and its benefits for managing cravings, reducing the intensity of urges, and breaking the cycle of substance use triggers.
2. **Identifying Distraction Strategies:** Brainstorm a list of distraction techniques and activities that can be used to shift focus away from cravings and urges, such as engaging in hobbies, physical exercise, or mindfulness practices.
3. **Creating a Distraction Plan:** Develop a personalized distraction plan outlining specific distraction techniques to use when faced with cravings or triggers, including alternative activities, coping skills, and support resources.
4. **Practice Distraction Techniques:** Practice implementing distraction techniques in simulated or imagined craving scenarios, experimenting with different strategies to identify what works best.
5. **Reflective Journaling:** Prompt participants to journal about their experience with distraction

techniques, noting any changes in cravings, mood, or behavior observed during the practice.

Guidance: Use this worksheet to introduce distraction techniques as a strategy for managing cravings and shifting focus away from substance use triggers. Focus on understanding distraction, identifying distraction strategies, creating a distraction plan, practicing distraction techniques, and reflecting on experiences.

Therapist Tips:

- Encourage participants to experiment with a variety of distraction techniques to identify what works best for them in managing cravings and shifting focus away from substance use triggers.
- Remind participants that distraction is a temporary coping strategy and may not eliminate cravings entirely, but can help reduce their intensity and duration.
- Offer guidance and support as participants explore distraction techniques, providing validation and encouragement of their efforts to develop effective coping skills in recovery.

Thought Stopping Technique

Description: This worksheet introduces the thought stopping technique as a strategy for interrupting and replacing intrusive or negative thoughts related to substance use.

Time: Allocate 15-20 minutes for this activity.

Activities:

1. **Understanding Thought Stopping:** Explain the concept of thought stopping and its benefits for managing intrusive or negative thoughts associated with substance use.
2. **Identifying Triggering Thoughts:** Help participants identify triggering thoughts or cognitive distortions that contribute to cravings or urges to use substances.
3. **Interrupting Negative Thoughts:** Teach participants how to use the thought stopping technique to interrupt and replace negative thoughts with more positive or neutral alternatives.
4. **Practice Thought Stopping:** Guide participants through a practice session where they actively apply the thought stopping technique to intrusive or negative thoughts related to substance use.
5. **Reflective Journaling:** Prompt participants to journal about their experience with the thought stopping technique, noting any changes in thought patterns, emotions, or cravings observed during the practice.

Guidance: Use this worksheet to introduce the thought stopping technique as a strategy for managing intrusive or negative thoughts related to substance use. Focus on understanding thought stopping, identifying triggering thoughts, interrupting negative thoughts, practicing the technique, and reflecting on experiences.

Therapist Tips:

- Encourage participants to practice the thought stopping technique regularly, especially when they notice intrusive or negative thoughts related to substance use.
- Remind participants that thought stopping is a skill that improves with practice, and it may take time to master the technique effectively.
- Offer guidance and support as participants explore the thought stopping technique, providing validation and encouragement of their efforts to challenge and change negative thought patterns in recovery.

Coping Cards

Description: This worksheet helps individuals create coping cards containing personalized coping strategies, affirmations, and reminders to use during times of stress or cravings.

Time: Set aside 15-20 minutes for this activity.

Activities:

1. **Identifying Coping Strategies:** Brainstorm a list of coping strategies and techniques that have been effective in managing stress or cravings in the past.

2. **Creating Coping Cards:** Encourage participants to write down their chosen coping strategies, affirmations, and reminders on index cards or small pieces of paper.

3. **Personalizing Coping Cards:** Have participants personalize their coping cards with colorful designs, drawings, or symbols that resonate with them.

4. **Keeping Coping Cards Accessible:** Instruct participants to keep their coping cards in easily accessible places, such as wallets, purses, or pockets, for quick reference during times of need.

5. **Reflective Journaling:** Prompt participants to journal about their experience creating coping cards, noting any feelings of empowerment, reassurance, or preparedness generated by the exercise.

Guidance: Use this worksheet to help individuals create coping cards containing personalized coping strategies, affirmations, and reminders to use during times of stress or cravings. Focus on identifying coping strategies, creating coping cards, personalizing them, keeping them accessible, and reflecting on the experience.

Therapist Tips:

*   Encourage participants to review their coping cards regularly, especially during challenging moments or when experiencing cravings or stress.
*   Remind participants that coping cards serve as portable reminders of their strengths, strategies,

and support systems, empowering them to navigate difficult situations effectively.

- Offer guidance and support as participants create and use coping cards, providing validation and encouragement of their efforts to develop personalized coping tools in recovery.

Social Support Network Mapping

Description: This worksheet helps individuals identify and visualize their social support network, including friends, family members, therapists, support groups, and other sources of support in their recovery journey.

Time: Allocate 20-30 minutes for this activity.

Activities:

1. **Identifying Supportive Individuals:** Prompt participants to list individuals who provide support, understanding, and encouragement in their recovery from substance abuse.
2. **Mapping the Support Network:** Have participants create a visual map or diagram of their social support network, connecting individuals with lines or arrows to represent relationships and connections.
3. **Assessing Support Levels:** Encourage participants to assess the level of support provided by each individual in their network, considering factors such as availability, reliability, and understanding.

4. **Identifying Gaps and Needs:** Help participants identify any gaps or areas where additional support may be needed in their social support network.
5. **Reflective Journaling:** Prompt participants to journal about their experience with social support network mapping, noting any insights, strengths, or challenges observed during the activity.

Guidance: Use this worksheet to help individuals identify and visualize their social support network, recognizing the importance of supportive relationships in their recovery journey. Focus on identifying supportive individuals, mapping the support network, assessing support levels, identifying gaps, and reflecting on the experience.

Therapist Tips:

- Encourage participants to reach out to supportive individuals in their network regularly, especially during times of need or when facing challenges in recovery.
- Remind participants that social support networks can evolve over time, and it's important to cultivate and nurture supportive relationships in recovery.
- Offer guidance and support as participants explore their social support network, providing validation and encouragement of their efforts to build a strong support system in recovery.

Relapse Analysis

Description: This worksheet helps individuals analyze the factors and triggers that contributed to a relapse, identify warning signs, and develop strategies to prevent future relapses.

Time: Set aside 20-30 minutes for this activity.

Activities:

1. **Reviewing the Relapse Event:** Prompt participants to recall and describe the circumstances, thoughts, emotions, and behaviors leading up to the relapse event.
2. **Identifying Triggers and Warning Signs:** Help participants identify the triggers, stressors, or situations that preceded the relapse, as well as any warning signs or red flags that indicated increased vulnerability to relapse.
3. **Analyzing Thoughts and Behaviors:** Encourage participants to analyze their thoughts, beliefs, and behaviors leading up to the relapse, identifying any cognitive distortions or maladaptive coping strategies.
4. **Developing Prevention Strategies:** Guide participants in developing personalized relapse prevention strategies, including coping skills, support systems, and lifestyle changes to address identified triggers and warning signs.

5. **Creating a Relapse Prevention Plan:** Assist participants in creating a written relapse prevention plan outlining specific strategies, coping skills, and support resources to prevent future relapses.

Guidance: Use this worksheet to help individuals analyze a relapse event, identify triggers and warning signs, and develop strategies to prevent future relapses. Focus on reviewing the relapse event, identifying triggers and warning signs, analyzing thoughts and behaviors, developing prevention strategies, and creating a relapse prevention plan.

Therapist Tips:

- Encourage participants to approach relapse analysis with self-compassion and curiosity, focusing on learning and growth rather than self-blame or judgment.
- Remind participants that relapse is a common and often expected part of the recovery process, and it provides valuable information for strengthening their relapse prevention strategies.
- Offer guidance and support as participants analyze their relapse event and develop a relapse prevention plan, providing validation and encouragement of their efforts to maintain sobriety and prevent future relapses.

Self-Efficacy Assessment

Description: This worksheet helps individuals assess their self-efficacy, or belief in their ability to resist cravings, cope with stress, and maintain sobriety in challenging situations.

Time: Allocate 15-20 minutes for this activity.

Activities:

1. **Defining Self-Efficacy:** Explain the concept of self-efficacy and its importance in recovery from substance abuse.
2. **Self-Efficacy Scale:** Have participants rate their confidence levels in resisting cravings, coping with stress, and maintaining sobriety in various situations using a self-efficacy scale (e.g., from 0% to 100%).
3. **Identifying Strengths and Weaknesses:** Prompt participants to reflect on their self-efficacy ratings and identify situations or triggers where their confidence is highest or lowest.
4. **Exploring Factors Affecting Self-Efficacy:** Discuss factors that may influence self-efficacy, such as past experiences, social support, coping skills, and beliefs about addiction and recovery.
5. **Setting Self-Efficacy Goals:** Help participants set realistic and achievable goals for increasing their self-efficacy in specific areas of recovery.

Guidance: Use this worksheet to help individuals assess their self-efficacy and develop strategies for increasing confidence in their ability to cope with cravings, stress, and challenges in recovery. Focus on defining self-efficacy, using a self-efficacy scale, identifying strengths and weaknesses, exploring influencing factors, and setting self-efficacy goals.

Therapist Tips:

- Encourage participants to focus on their strengths and past successes in recovery when assessing their self-efficacy.
- Remind participants that self-efficacy can be cultivated and strengthened through practice, support, and positive reinforcement.
- Offer guidance and support as participants reflect on their self-efficacy and set goals for increasing confidence in recovery, providing validation and encouragement of their efforts to build self-efficacy.

Time Management Planning

Description: This worksheet helps individuals develop effective time management skills to prioritize recovery-related activities, responsibilities, and goals.

Time: Set aside 20-30 minutes for this activity.

Activities:

1. **Identifying Recovery Priorities:** Prompt participants to identify and prioritize recovery-related activities, responsibilities, and goals, such

as attending therapy sessions, engaging in support groups, and practicing coping skills.

2. **Creating a Weekly Schedule:** Assist participants in creating a weekly schedule or planner, allocating time slots for recovery activities, work or school commitments, self-care, and leisure activities.

3. **Setting SMART Goals:** Encourage participants to set specific, measurable, achievable, relevant, and time-bound (SMART) goals related to their recovery, breaking larger goals into smaller, manageable tasks.

4. **Balancing Responsibilities:** Help participants balance recovery-related activities with other responsibilities and commitments, ensuring they allocate sufficient time and energy for self-care and relaxation.

5. **Monitoring Progress:** Encourage participants to regularly review and update their weekly schedule, tracking progress toward their goals and making adjustments as needed.

Guidance: Use this worksheet to help individuals develop effective time management skills to prioritize recovery-related activities and responsibilities. Focus on identifying priorities, creating a weekly schedule, setting SMART goals, balancing responsibilities, and monitoring progress.

Therapist Tips:

- Encourage participants to be realistic and flexible when planning their schedules, allowing for unexpected events or changes in priorities.
- Remind participants that effective time management can help reduce stress, increase productivity, and enhance overall well-being in recovery.
- Offer guidance and support as participants develop their time management skills, providing validation and encouragement of their efforts to prioritize recovery and achieve their goals.

Assertiveness Training

Description: This worksheet introduces assertiveness training as a strategy for effectively communicating needs, setting boundaries, and advocating for oneself in recovery.

Time: Allocate 20-30 minutes for this activity.

Activities:

1. **Understanding Assertiveness:** Explain the concept of assertiveness and its importance in recovery from substance abuse, emphasizing the difference between passive, aggressive, and assertive communication styles.
2. **Identifying Assertive Communication Skills:** Discuss key assertive communication skills, such as using "I" statements, expressing feelings and needs clearly, and standing up for oneself while respecting others.

3. **Role-Playing Scenarios:** Engage participants in role-playing exercises where they practice assertive communication skills in various recovery-related scenarios, such as refusing offers of alcohol or drugs, setting boundaries with friends or family members, and asking for support or assistance.

4. **Assertiveness Training Techniques:** Teach participants specific assertiveness training techniques, such as broken record technique, fogging, and negative assertion, to handle challenging situations with confidence and self-assurance.

5. **Reflective Journaling:** Prompt participants to journal about their experience with assertiveness training, noting any insights, challenges, or successes observed during the exercises.

Guidance: Use this worksheet to introduce assertiveness training as a strategy for effectively communicating needs, setting boundaries, and advocating for oneself in recovery. Focus on understanding assertiveness, identifying assertive communication skills, practicing role-playing scenarios, learning assertiveness training techniques, and reflecting on experiences.

Therapist Tips:

- Encourage participants to practice assertive communication skills regularly, both in role-playing exercises and real-life situations, to build confidence and competence over time.

- Remind participants that assertiveness is a skill that can be learned and developed with practice, and it is essential for maintaining healthy relationships and boundaries in recovery.
- Offer guidance and support as participants engage in assertiveness training exercises, providing validation and encouragement of their efforts to communicate assertively and advocate for their needs in recovery.

Coping Skills Toolbox

Description: This worksheet helps individuals create a personalized coping skills toolbox containing a variety of strategies and techniques to manage cravings, cope with stress, and navigate challenges in recovery.

Time: Allocate 20-30 minutes for this activity.

Activities:

1. **Identifying Coping Skills:** Prompt participants to brainstorm a list of coping skills and techniques they have found helpful in managing cravings, stress, and difficult emotions. This can include activities like deep breathing, mindfulness meditation, journaling, exercise, and reaching out to a supportive friend.
2. **Creating a Coping Skills Toolbox:** Provide participants with a template or worksheet where they can organize their coping skills into categories (e.g., relaxation techniques, distraction strategies,

social support resources) and create a personalized coping skills toolbox.

3. **Exploring Coping Strategies:** Encourage participants to explore new coping strategies and techniques they may not have tried before, such as progressive muscle relaxation, guided imagery, or grounding exercises.

4. **Practicing Coping Skills:** Prompt participants to practice using their coping skills toolbox regularly, especially during times of stress, cravings, or emotional distress. Encourage them to experiment with different techniques to find what works best for them.

5. **Reflective Journaling:** Encourage participants to journal about their experiences using coping skills from their toolbox, noting which strategies were most effective in different situations and any insights or observations gained from the practice.

Guidance: Use this worksheet to help individuals create a personalized coping skills toolbox containing a variety of strategies and techniques to manage cravings, cope with stress, and navigate challenges in recovery. Focus on identifying coping skills, organizing them into a toolbox, exploring new strategies, practicing coping skills, and reflecting on experiences.

Therapist Tips:

- Encourage participants to be creative and open-minded when brainstorming coping skills for their toolbox, considering a diverse range of techniques that resonate with them personally.

- Remind participants that building a coping skills toolbox is an ongoing process, and it's okay to add or remove strategies as needed based on their effectiveness and relevance to their current needs.
- Offer guidance and support as participants explore and practice coping skills from their toolbox, providing validation and encouragement of their efforts to develop healthy coping strategies in recovery.

Practical Scenarios

Practical Scenarios" section serves as a bridge between theory and practice, helping readers translate theoretical knowledge into actionable strategies they can use to overcome real-life challenges on their journey to sobriety.

Sarah's Recovery Journey

Sarah, a 28-year-old marketing executive, has been struggling with substance abuse for several years. She primarily abuses alcohol as a way to cope with stress and anxiety related to her demanding job. After hitting rock bottom and experiencing a series of negative consequences due to her alcohol use, including strained relationships and declining mental health, Sarah decides to seek help and embark on a journey to recovery.

Application of Section 1: Self-Reflection

Sarah begins her recovery journey by engaging in self-reflection worksheets from the book "Worksheets for Substance Abuse." She takes time to reflect on her past experiences with alcohol, identifying triggers such as work-related stress, social gatherings, and feelings of loneliness. Through guided exercises, Sarah gains insight into the underlying emotions and thought patterns driving her substance abuse.

Application of Section 2: Goal Setting and Action Plans

With a clearer understanding of her triggers and motivations, Sarah sets specific goals for her recovery. Using goal-setting worksheets, she outlines actionable steps, including attending therapy sessions, joining a support group, and developing healthier coping strategies like exercise and mindfulness meditation. Sarah creates a detailed action plan to achieve her goals, breaking down each step into manageable tasks.

Application of Section 3: Coping Strategies

As Sarah progresses in her recovery journey, she encounters challenges and cravings for alcohol. Drawing on coping strategies worksheets, she implements techniques such as deep breathing exercises, mindfulness meditation, and reaching out to supportive friends and family members. Sarah also practices assertiveness training exercises to communicate her needs effectively and set boundaries in her relationships.

Application of Section 4: Cognitive-Behavioral Techniques

Despite her efforts, Sarah experiences negative thoughts and self-doubt along the way. Using cognitive-behavioral techniques worksheets, she learns to challenge these irrational beliefs and reframe them in a more positive light. Sarah keeps a thought record to track her thoughts and emotions, identifying patterns and learning to replace negative thoughts with more constructive ones.

Application of Section 5: Relapse Prevention Strategies

As Sarah approaches a critical juncture in her recovery, she focuses on relapse prevention strategies to maintain her sobriety. She creates a relapse prevention plan, identifying warning signs such as increased stress and social isolation. Sarah develops emergency coping strategies to navigate these situations effectively, such as reaching out to her sponsor or engaging in alternative activities to distract herself from cravings.

Conclusion and Ongoing Support:

Sarah's journey to recovery is a testament to the transformative power of the resources provided in "Worksheets for Substance Abuse." By engaging in self-reflection, setting goals, practicing coping strategies, utilizing cognitive-behavioral techniques, and implementing relapse prevention strategies, Sarah achieves significant progress in her recovery. However, her journey doesn't end here. Sarah continues to use the worksheets and resources from the book as ongoing support in her recovery journey, attending therapy sessions, participating in support groups, and accessing additional resources as needed. With dedication, perseverance, and the right tools, Sarah is able to overcome her substance abuse and build a healthier, happier life for herself.

David's Path to Sobriety

David, a 42-year-old construction worker, has struggled with opioid addiction for over a decade. His addiction began after a work-related injury led to a prescription for painkillers, which eventually spiraled into substance abuse. Despite numerous attempts to quit on his own, David finds himself trapped in a cycle of addiction, unable to break free. After hitting rock bottom and experiencing the loss of his job and strained relationships with his family, David realizes he needs help and decides to seek treatment.

Application of Section 1: Self-Reflection

Upon entering a rehabilitation program, David is introduced to the self-reflection worksheets from "Worksheets for Substance Abuse." Through these exercises, David reflects on his past experiences with opioids, identifying triggers such as chronic pain, stress, and social isolation. He delves deep into his emotions and thought patterns, gaining insight into the underlying reasons for his substance abuse.

Application of Section 2: Goal Setting and Action Plans

With newfound clarity, David sets specific goals for his recovery journey. Using the goal-setting worksheets, he outlines actionable steps, including attending therapy sessions, participating in a support group, and exploring alternative pain management techniques such as physical therapy and acupuncture. David develops a comprehensive action plan to achieve his goals, breaking down each step into manageable tasks.

Application of Section 3: Coping Strategies

As David progresses in his recovery, he encounters challenges and cravings for opioids. Leveraging the coping strategies worksheets, he implements techniques such as mindfulness meditation, deep breathing exercises, and journaling to manage his cravings and cope with stress. David also learns assertiveness training to communicate his needs effectively and establish healthy boundaries in his relationships.

Application of Section 4: Cognitive-Behavioral Techniques

Despite his efforts, David struggles with negative thoughts and self-doubt throughout his recovery journey. Using the cognitive-behavioral techniques worksheets, he learns to challenge these thoughts and reframe them in a more positive light. David keeps a thought journal to track his progress and identify patterns, replacing negative thoughts with affirmations and positive affirmations.

Application of Section 5: Relapse Prevention Strategies

As David nears the completion of his rehabilitation program, he focuses on relapse prevention strategies to maintain his sobriety in the long term. He creates a relapse prevention plan, identifying triggers such as chronic pain flare-ups and stressful situations. David develops coping strategies to navigate these triggers, such as reaching out to his support network, engaging in hobbies, and seeking professional help if needed.

Conclusion and Ongoing Support:

David's journey to sobriety is a testament to the effectiveness of the resources provided in "Worksheets for Substance Abuse." Through self-reflection, goal setting, coping strategies, cognitive-behavioral techniques, and relapse prevention strategies, David makes significant strides in his recovery. However, his journey doesn't end here. David continues to utilize the worksheets and resources from the book as ongoing support in his journey to sobriety, attending therapy sessions, participating in support groups, and accessing additional resources as needed. With determination, perseverance, and the right tools, David is able to overcome his opioid addiction and reclaim his life.

Emily's Journey to Overcoming Cocaine Addiction

Emily, a 30-year-old graphic designer, has been battling cocaine addiction for several years. Her addiction began during college, where she turned to cocaine as a way to cope with academic stress and social anxiety. Despite several attempts to quit using on her own, Emily finds herself caught in a cycle of addiction, leading to strained relationships and declining mental health. Determined to regain control of her life, Emily decides to seek professional help and embark on a journey to recovery.

Application of Section 1: Self-Reflection

Upon entering a residential rehabilitation facility, Emily begins working through the self-reflection worksheets provided in "Worksheets for Substance Abuse." Through these exercises, Emily reflects on her past experiences with cocaine, identifying triggers such as social gatherings, feelings of inadequacy, and moments of boredom. She explores the emotions and thought patterns underlying her substance abuse, gaining insight into the root causes of her addiction.

Application of Section 2: Goal Setting and Action Plans

With a better understanding of her triggers and motivations, Emily sets specific goals for her recovery. Using the goal-setting worksheets, she outlines actionable steps, including attending counseling sessions, participating in recreational activities that promote sobriety, and reconnecting with supportive friends and family members. Emily creates a detailed action plan to achieve her goals, breaking down each step into manageable tasks.

Application of Section 3: Coping Strategies

As Emily progresses in her recovery, she encounters challenges and cravings for cocaine. Utilizing the coping strategies worksheets, she implements techniques such as mindfulness meditation, engaging in creative outlets like painting and writing, and practicing relaxation exercises to manage her cravings and cope with stress. Emily also learns assertiveness training to communicate her needs effectively and set boundaries in her relationships.

Application of Section 4: Cognitive-Behavioral Techniques

Despite her efforts, Emily grapples with negative thoughts and self-doubt throughout her recovery journey. Using the cognitive-behavioral techniques worksheets, she learns to challenge these thoughts and reframe them in a more positive light. Emily keeps a thought journal to track her progress and identify patterns, replacing negative thoughts with affirmations and positive self-talk.

Application of Section 5: Relapse Prevention Strategies

As Emily nears the end of her residential program, she focuses on relapse prevention strategies to maintain her sobriety in the long term. She creates a relapse prevention plan, identifying triggers such as stressors related to work deadlines and social pressures. Emily develops coping strategies to navigate these triggers, such as reaching out to her support network, engaging in healthy activities, and attending regular therapy sessions.

Conclusion and Ongoing Support:

Emily's journey to overcoming cocaine addiction demonstrates the transformative impact of the resources provided in "Worksheets for Substance Abuse." Through self-reflection, goal setting, coping strategies, cognitive-behavioral techniques, and relapse prevention strategies, Emily makes significant progress in her recovery. However, her journey doesn't end here. Emily continues to utilize the worksheets and resources from the book as ongoing support in her journey to sobriety, attending therapy sessions, participating in support groups, and accessing additional resources as needed. With perseverance and the right tools, Emily is able to break free from the grip of addiction and build a brighter future for herself.

Michael's Recovery from Marijuana Addiction

Michael, a 25-year-old college graduate, has been struggling with marijuana addiction since his teenage years. Initially, he started using marijuana recreationally with friends, but over time, it escalated into a daily habit to cope with stress and anxiety. Despite recognizing the negative impact on his relationships, academics, and mental health, Michael found it difficult to quit on his own. Realizing he needed help, Michael decides to enroll in an outpatient rehabilitation program to address his addiction.

Application of Section 1: Self-Reflection

At the beginning of his rehabilitation journey, Michael engages in self-reflection worksheets to explore his relationship with marijuana. Through these exercises, he identifies triggers such as social situations, boredom, and negative emotions like anxiety and depression. By delving into his past experiences and thought patterns, Michael gains insight into the underlying reasons for his substance use.

Application of Section 2: Goal Setting and Action Plans

With a clearer understanding of his triggers and motivations, Michael sets specific goals for his recovery. Using goal-setting worksheets, he outlines actionable steps, including attending counseling sessions, finding alternative ways to manage stress such as exercise and meditation, and reconnecting with hobbies and interests he enjoyed before his addiction. Michael creates a structured action plan to implement these changes into his daily life.

Application of Section 3: Coping Strategies

As Michael progresses in his recovery, he encounters cravings and challenges associated with quitting marijuana. Leveraging coping strategies worksheets, he practices techniques such as mindfulness meditation, deep breathing exercises, and engaging in activities that bring him joy and fulfillment. Michael also learns to identify and challenge negative thought patterns that contribute to his cravings, replacing them with more positive and empowering thoughts.

Application of Section 4: Cognitive-Behavioral Techniques

Throughout his journey, Michael works on cognitive-behavioral techniques to address underlying issues contributing to his addiction. Using worksheets focused on cognitive restructuring and thought records, he learns to challenge irrational beliefs about marijuana and understand the consequences of his substance use. By reframing his thoughts and developing healthier coping mechanisms, Michael gains confidence in his ability to overcome his addiction.

Application of Section 5: Relapse Prevention Strategies

As Michael nears the completion of his rehabilitation program, he focuses on relapse prevention strategies to maintain his sobriety in the long term. He creates a relapse prevention plan, identifying potential triggers such as stress, peer pressure, and social gatherings where marijuana may be present. Michael develops coping strategies to navigate these triggers, such as reaching out to his support network, attending support group meetings, and practicing self-care activities to manage stress effectively.

Conclusion and Ongoing Support:

Michael's journey to recovery from marijuana addiction showcases the effectiveness of the resources provided in "Worksheets for Substance Abuse." Through self-reflection, goal setting, coping strategies, cognitive-behavioral techniques, and relapse prevention strategies, Michael makes significant progress in overcoming his addiction. However, his journey doesn't end here. Michael continues to utilize the worksheets and resources from the book as ongoing support in his journey to sobriety, attending follow-up therapy sessions, participating in support groups, and implementing healthy lifestyle changes to maintain his progress. With dedication and perseverance, Michael is able to break free from the cycle of addiction and build a fulfilling life in recovery.

Top of Form

Sarah's Recovery Journey from Alcohol Addiction

Sarah, a 35-year-old teacher, has been struggling with alcohol addiction for several years. What started as occasional social drinking to unwind gradually escalated into a daily habit to cope with stress and personal challenges. Despite recognizing the negative impact of alcohol on her health, career, and relationships, Sarah found it difficult to quit on her own. After a particularly embarrassing incident at a school event, Sarah decides to seek professional help and enroll in a residential rehabilitation program.

Application of Section 1: Self-Reflection

Upon entering the rehabilitation facility, Sarah begins her journey to recovery by engaging in self-reflection worksheets. Through these exercises, she explores her relationship with alcohol, identifying triggers such as work-related stress, social gatherings, and feelings of loneliness. By delving into her past experiences and emotional triggers, Sarah gains insight into the underlying reasons for her substance use.

Application of Section 2: Goal Setting and Action Plans

With a newfound understanding of her triggers and motivations, Sarah sets specific goals for her recovery. Using goal-setting worksheets, she outlines actionable steps, including attending daily therapy sessions, participating in group counseling, and practicing mindfulness techniques to manage cravings. Sarah creates a structured action plan to implement these changes into her daily routine.

Application of Section 3: Coping Strategies

As Sarah progresses in her recovery, she encounters challenges and cravings associated with quitting alcohol. Leveraging coping strategies worksheets, she practices techniques such as deep breathing exercises, journaling, and engaging in hobbies that bring her joy. Sarah also learns to identify and challenge negative thought patterns that contribute to her cravings, replacing them with positive affirmations and self-care practices.

Application of Section 4: Cognitive-Behavioral Techniques

Throughout her rehabilitation journey, Sarah works on cognitive-behavioral techniques to address underlying issues contributing to her addiction. Using worksheets focused on cognitive restructuring and thought records, she learns to challenge irrational beliefs about alcohol and understand the consequences of her substance use. By reframing her thoughts and developing healthier coping mechanisms, Sarah gains confidence in her ability to overcome her addiction.

Application of Section 5: Relapse Prevention Strategies

As Sarah nears the end of her residential program, she focuses on relapse prevention strategies to maintain her sobriety in the long term. She creates a relapse prevention plan, identifying potential triggers such as stress, social events, and emotional distress. Sarah develops coping strategies to navigate these triggers, such as reaching out to her support network, attending Alcoholics Anonymous meetings, and practicing self-care activities to manage stress effectively.

Conclusion and Ongoing Support:

Sarah's journey to recovery from alcohol addiction demonstrates the transformative power of the resources provided in "Worksheets for Substance Abuse." Through self-reflection, goal setting, coping strategies, cognitive-behavioral techniques, and relapse prevention strategies, Sarah makes significant progress in overcoming her addiction. However, her journey doesn't end here. Sarah continues to utilize the worksheets and resources from the book as ongoing support in her journey to sobriety, attending outpatient therapy sessions, participating in support groups, and implementing healthy lifestyle changes to maintain her progress. With dedication and perseverance, Sarah is able to break free from the grip of alcohol addiction and build a fulfilling life in recovery.

Alex's Journey to Overcoming Prescription Drug Addiction

Alex, a 28-year-old marketing executive, has been struggling with prescription drug addiction for several years. It all began innocently after a sports injury led to a prescription for painkillers. Over time, Alex's occasional use escalated into dependence as he found himself relying on the medication to cope with stress and manage chronic pain. Despite recognizing the negative impact on his health, career, and relationships, Alex struggled to break free from the grip of addiction. After a wake-up call from a close friend expressing concern about his well-being, Alex decides to seek professional help and enters an intensive outpatient rehabilitation program.

Application of Section 1: Self-Reflection

At the start of his rehabilitation journey, Alex engages in self-reflection worksheets to explore his relationship with prescription drugs. Through these exercises, he identifies triggers such as physical pain, work-related stress, and feelings of inadequacy. By delving into his past experiences and emotional triggers, Alex gains insight into the underlying reasons for his substance use.

Application of Section 2: Goal Setting and Action Plans

With a clearer understanding of his triggers and motivations, Alex sets specific goals for his recovery. Using goal-setting worksheets, he outlines actionable steps, including attending therapy sessions, participating in alternative pain management techniques such as physical therapy and acupuncture, and rebuilding his social support network. Alex creates a structured action plan to implement these changes into his daily routine.

Application of Section 3: Coping Strategies

As Alex progresses in his recovery, he encounters challenges and cravings associated with quitting prescription drugs. Leveraging coping strategies worksheets, he practices techniques such as mindfulness meditation, deep breathing exercises, and engaging in hobbies that distract him from his cravings. Alex also learns to identify and challenge negative thought patterns that contribute to his substance use, replacing them with positive affirmations and self-care practices.

Application of Section 4: Cognitive-Behavioral Techniques

Throughout his rehabilitation journey, Alex works on cognitive-behavioral techniques to address underlying issues contributing to his addiction. Using worksheets focused on cognitive restructuring and thought records, he learns to challenge irrational beliefs about prescription drugs and understand the consequences of his substance use. By reframing his thoughts and developing healthier coping mechanisms, Alex gains confidence in his ability to overcome his addiction.

Application of Section 5: Relapse Prevention Strategies

As Alex nears the completion of his outpatient program, he focuses on relapse prevention strategies to maintain his sobriety in the long term. He creates a relapse prevention plan, identifying potential triggers such as physical pain flare-ups and work-related stressors. Alex develops coping strategies to navigate these triggers, such as reaching out to his support network, attending support group meetings, and practicing self-care activities to manage stress effectively.

Conclusion and Ongoing Support:

Alex's journey to recovery from prescription drug addiction exemplifies the transformative impact of the resources provided in "Worksheets for Substance Abuse." Through self-reflection, goal setting, coping strategies, cognitive-behavioral techniques, and relapse prevention strategies, Alex makes significant progress in overcoming his addiction. However, his journey doesn't end here. Alex continues to utilize the worksheets and resources from the book as ongoing support in his journey to sobriety, attending follow-up therapy sessions, participating in support groups, and implementing healthy lifestyle changes to maintain his progress. With determination and perseverance, Alex is able to reclaim his life from the clutches of addiction and build a brighter future for himself.

Emily's Struggle with Methamphetamine Addiction

Emily, a 30-year-old graphic designer, has been grappling with methamphetamine addiction for the past five years. What started as experimental use during college parties quickly spiraled into a full-blown addiction as Emily sought to escape from the pressures of work and strained relationships. Despite multiple attempts to quit cold turkey, Emily found herself trapped in a cycle of relapse and despair. Faced with mounting consequences, including job loss and strained family ties, Emily realizes she needs professional help and seeks admission to an inpatient rehabilitation facility.

Application of Section 1: Self-Reflection

Upon admission to the rehabilitation facility, Emily begins her journey to recovery by engaging in self-reflection worksheets. Through introspection, she identifies triggers such as work stress, relationship conflicts, and feelings of low self-worth. By delving into her past experiences and emotional triggers, Emily gains insight into the root causes of her substance use.

Application of Section 2: Goal Setting and Action Plans

With newfound clarity, Emily sets specific goals for her recovery using worksheets provided in the rehabilitation program. She commits to attending therapy sessions, participating in group counseling, and rebuilding her life outside of addiction. Emily creates a detailed action plan, outlining steps to reconnect with sober friends, pursue hobbies she once enjoyed, and develop healthier coping mechanisms to manage stress.

Application of Section 3: Coping Strategies

As Emily progresses in her recovery journey, she learns and practices coping strategies to navigate cravings and challenging emotions. Using worksheets focused on coping techniques, Emily engages in mindfulness exercises, practices assertive communication, and learns to challenge negative thought patterns. With support from her therapists and peers, Emily begins to replace destructive behaviors with healthier alternatives.

Application of Section 4: Cognitive-Behavioral Techniques

Emily delves deeper into cognitive-behavioral techniques to address the underlying issues fueling her addiction. Through worksheets focused on cognitive restructuring and thought records, she learns to challenge distorted thinking patterns and reframe her perceptions of herself and the world around her. Emily discovers the power of positive self-talk and begins to cultivate a more compassionate and resilient mindset.

Application of Section 5: Relapse Prevention Strategies

As Emily nears the end of her inpatient program, she focuses on developing relapse prevention strategies to maintain her sobriety in the face of challenges. She creates a comprehensive relapse prevention plan, identifying potential triggers such as stress, boredom, and social isolation. Emily equips herself with coping skills to manage cravings, including reaching out to her support network, attending recovery meetings, and engaging in healthy activities that bring her joy and fulfillment.

Conclusion and Ongoing Support:

Emily's journey to recovery from methamphetamine addiction exemplifies the transformative impact of rehabilitation resources. Through self-reflection, goal setting, coping strategies, cognitive-behavioral techniques, and relapse prevention strategies, Emily makes significant strides in overcoming her addiction. However, her journey continues beyond the confines of the rehabilitation facility. Emily commits to ongoing therapy, participation in support groups, and the continued use of recovery worksheets to maintain her progress and build a fulfilling life free from the shackles of addiction. With determination and support,

Emily embarks on a new chapter filled with hope, resilience, and a renewed sense of purpose.

References

1. Substance Abuse and Mental Health Services Administration (SAMHSA). (2016). Treatment Improvement Protocol (TIP) Series, No. 34. Rockville, MD: Center for Substance Abuse Treatment.

2. National Institute on Drug Abuse (NIDA). (2020). Principles of Drug Addiction Treatment: A Research-Based Guide (Third Edition). Bethesda, MD: National Institutes of Health.

3. Gorski, T., & Miller, M. (2018). Staying Sober: A Guide for Relapse Prevention. Independence, MO: Herald House/Independence Press.

4. Marlatt, G. A., & Donovan, D. M. (Eds.). (2005). Relapse Prevention: Maintenance Strategies in the Treatment of Addictive Behaviors (2nd ed.). New York, NY: The Guilford Press.

5. Hayes, S. C., Strosahl, K. D., & Wilson, K. G. (2011). Acceptance and Commitment Therapy: The Process and Practice of Mindful Change (2nd ed.). New York, NY: The Guilford Press.

6. Najavits, L. M. (2002). Seeking Safety: A Treatment Manual for PTSD and Substance Abuse. New York, NY: The Guilford Press.

7. Prochaska, J. O., & Norcross, J. C. (2018). Systems of Psychotherapy: A Transtheoretical Analysis (9th ed.). Oxford, UK: Oxford University Press.

8. Center for Substance Abuse Treatment. (2006). Substance Abuse Treatment: Addressing the

Specific Needs of Women. Rockville, MD: Substance
Abuse and Mental Health Services Administration.

9. Kadden, R. M., & Carroll, K. M. (2001). Cognitive-
Behavioral Coping Skills Therapy Manual: A Clinical
Research Guide for Therapists Treating Individuals
With Alcohol Abuse and Dependence (Vol. 3).
Rockville, MD: National Institute on Alcohol Abuse
and Alcoholism.

10. Dimeff, L. A., & Linehan, M. M. (2008). Dialectical
Behavior Therapy for Substance Abusers. New York,
NY: The Guilford Press.

www.ingramcontent.com/pod-product-compliance
Lightning Source LLC
Chambersburg PA
CBHW062208270326
41930CB00009B/1677